HEALING PETS

With Nature's Miracle Cures

HEALING PETS

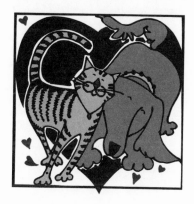

With Nature's Miracle Cures

Henry Pasternak, D.V.M., C.V.A.

Highlands Veterinary Hospital
Pacific Palisades, California

This book is dedicated
to all of my four-legged teachers.

Published by
Highlands Veterinary Hospital
526 Palisades Drive
Pacific Palisades, CA 90372
310-454-2917
310-454-3412 fax
E-mail: pupydoc@aol.com

ISBN 0-9709678-4-5
Library of Congress Control Number: 2001094320

Design & Editorial Services by The Roberts Group
Cover Design by Gemini Group

CONTENTS

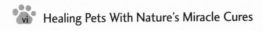

PREFACE

Healing Pets With Nature's Miracle Cures provides you with the intellectual foundation and tools to understand and make sense of holistic, as well as modern western techniques, used to maximize the body's natural healing abilities. For many years, I have practiced medicine combining the latest modern techniques with the wisdom of "holism." Many acute situations require the use of "invasive" procedures and measures to save lives, while chronic diseases respond better to "noninvasive" measures such as herbs, acupuncture, homeopathy, etc. We must remember that pain is not a deficiency of aspirin or prednisone, but an imbalance in the animal's terrain. If there is disease, it does not mean that we lack the latest chemotherapy drug or antibiotic, but rather that there is an imbalance in the body.

This book is about balance. Bacteria only cause infection when the biological terrain is out of balance. Bacteria take advantage of a body weakened by nutrient-poor food or burdened by toxins that don't belong in the biological system. While the latest antibiotics are indicated in the treatment of acute life-threatening infections, we also should be attempting to reestablish balance and stimulate the body's natural healing abilities.

The information in this book is intended as an educational tool to acquaint you with alternative methods for maintaining your pet's good health and treating its illnesses. Remember, that in the ideal partnership, both the pet owner and the veterinarian work together toward the goal of helping animal companions live healthy and happy lives.

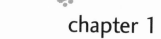

chapter 1

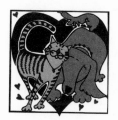 **Introduction:
Natural Methods Stress
Health Maintenance and
Disease Prevention**

A REVOLUTION IN THE HEALTHCARE SYSTEM FOR MAN AND ANIMAL is
now sweeping the globe. Science and medicine have the technology to understand and appreciate the value of integrating
"natural" and conventional therapies. The roots of natural
medicine can be traced back to the philosophy of Hippocrates.
This is a health-oriented system of medicine that stresses maintenance of health and prevention of disease. Conventional
medicine is superb in acute, emergency, and traumatic situations; I often use conventional medicine initially to stabilize
the patient. Then I always follow up with alternative medicine
for long-term treatment.

Holistic medicine is more cost-effective over the long term
because it seeks to treat the root of the problem and not only the
symptoms; it doesn't trap the patient on a merry-go-round that

begins with one drug and ends up requiring others to compensate for the side effects caused by the initial drugs. Many holistic methods work by assisting the body's own natural healing system instead of introducing strong drugs.

The fundamental philosophy of natural medicine is that the body has the ability to heal itself given the proper opportunity. For example, some herbs seem to have organ-specific actions and by implementing these herbs for certain diseases, the body may be able to heal much faster without side effects. Milk thistle is a good example of an herb used to treat liver disease. Certainly, bacterial infections require appropriate antibiotics; however, chronic infections can be cured much faster with good nutrition, herbs, acupuncture, homeopathic remedies, and other modalities.

After many years of veterinary practice, I have come to realize that although thousands of diseases have been named, only a relatively few imbalances cause them. The actual symptoms or disease that is manifested are determined by the underlying imbalance in the biological terrain.[1]

This book provides a step-by-step journey through each system of the body. Written in layman's terms, it offers a comprehensive yet understandable discussion of the key underlying systems in the body and what each system needs for optimum health. For each system of the body, I talk about how holistic and conventional medicine can work together effectively. No matter what form of medicine or treatment we choose for our pets, we must always remember to bring about the fastest effective cure without doing additional harm. Both pet owners and veterinarians must work together to ease an animal's pain and discomfort and put aside all prejudices as to which form of medicine is superior to the other. Optimum health can only be achieved when all forms of medicine are considered, and used, in appropriate situations.

This book provides practical healing methods for animals suffering from chronic disease and those that are constantly contracting one disease after another. Prevention of disease is just as important as treatment—this is the underlying theme of *Healing Pets With Nature's Miracle Cures.*

Though it is easy to prescribe a raw food diet, herbs, and exercise, the individual's unique situation must be taken into consideration. Dogs and cats have a tremendous ability to heal, usually without drug or herbal intervention. It is estimated that 70 to 80 percent of all diseases are self-limiting and will heal without drug or herbal intervention. Nature has marvelous healing abilities, and the symptoms that we are presented with should not be suppressed but studied so that a holistic approach to disease can be instituted to affect a permanent cure. When the body's natural healing system is overloaded, symptoms and disease situations result. If we only treat the symptoms instead of the underlying imbalance, the situation may result in chronic disease and susceptibility to a more serious situation in the future.

Homeostasis is when the body's internal environment balances the hazards of the external environment. For example, when the body is exposed to infectious organisms, the body mounts an aggressive defense response, which might be evidenced in fever. Unfortunately, rather than respecting these homeostatic processes and waiting for them to finish their task, many people actively try to suppress the symptoms of self-repair—whether this be a raised temperature or inflammation in an injured area. If homeostasis is to be maintained, it is important to recognize those symptoms as part of the normal healing process. Unless the animal is suffering or its life is in danger, the symptoms should be left alone so that the natural repair process can proceed unimpaired.

The intent of this book is to help pet owners understand the fundamentals of optimum health, the logic behind natural therapies, and when to seek professional advice. Some therapies, such as acupuncture or QiGong, which have been used successfully for thousands of years in China, are only now being explained with modern scientific methods. It is hoped that the scientific information provided in this book may bridge a dialogue between the pet owner and the veterinarian.

chapter 2

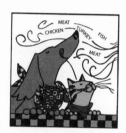

Nutrition: Which Food Should You Choose for Your Animal Companion?

THE IMAGES THAT PET FOOD MANUFACTURERS PROMULGATE—images of whole chicken, choice cuts of beef, fresh grains, vitamins, and minerals that meet all your pet's needs for a healthy existence—are a bit deceiving. What they don't tell you is that instead of whole chicken, manufacturers have substituted chicken heads, feet, intestines, and bowels. The choice cuts of beef have been replaced with cow brains, tongue, esophagus, ears, and any other part that is condemned for human consumption. Grains used in pet foods have not been tested for impurities such as mold or pesticides.

The pet food industry must "fortify" its products with vitamins and minerals to make sure the food is nutritious, since many nutrients are destroyed during the manufacturing process. In fact, much of the ingredients in pet foods are leftovers from the human food industry—food deemed not fit for human consumption. And yet, we are told by the pet food industry not to feed table scraps to our pets because doing so may somehow "unbalance" their nutrient intake. Scientists for the pet food industry have learned how to make questionable food palatable—food that, under ordinary circumstances, your pet would turn up its nose to.

The Pet Food Institute acknowledges the importance of using by-products in pet foods to provide additional income for processors and farmers.[1] Many of these remnants are indigestible and provide a questionable source of nutrition for dogs and cats. Furthermore, the amount of nutrition in meat by-products, meals, and animal fats varies from batch to batch. It stands to reason that a vat filled with chicken feet, beaks, and viscera is going to yield less digestible protein than a vat of breast meat. There is little or no information on the bio-availability of the nutrients in food manufactured for companion animals.[2] In other words, it is not known if and how those nutrients are absorbed by the animals' bodies. Nutrient profiles by the Association of American Feed Control Officials (AAFCO) do not give assurance of nutritional adequacy and will not until bio-availability values are known.

The well-known phrase, "meat by-products," is a misnomer since these by-products contain little, if any, meat. These are the parts of the animal left over after the meat has been stripped away from the bone. Chicken by-products include head, feet, entrails, lungs, spleen, kidneys, brain, liver, stomach, bones, blood, intestines, and any other part of the carcass not fit for human consumption. One of the dirty little secrets kept by the pet food industry is that some by-products also contain substances such as abscesses and cancerous material. In my opinion, feeding slaughterhouse wastes to animals increases their chances of getting cancer and other degenerative diseases. Some meat, especially glandular tissue, may contain high levels of hormones, which may also cause serious health problems including cancer. Unlike bacteria and viruses, these hormones are not destroyed by the high temperatures or pressure cooking used in the manufacture of pet food. Cats seem to be most adversely affected by high hormone levels.[3]

Pet food manufacturers have solved the problem of palatability by spraying fat or "digest" on kibble. The fat also acts as a binder for other flavor enhancers. Unfortunately, it creates another problem: rancidity. Rancid fat can accelerate free radical damage and cause a variety of diseases. To prevent rancidity, powerful antioxidants are added.

The canning process sterilizes and destroys all microbes, so we need not worry about salmonella or botulism. However, the high temperatures used to destroy the microbes also destroy the nutrients. To compensate for what has been lost during the cooking and canning process, pet food manufacturers add vitamins, minerals, and amino acids to their products. It has been shown, however, that these synthetic vitamins are not absorbed by the body as well as vitamins that occur through a natural diet.[4] I have always favored a wholesome raw diet over synthetic pills and concoctions. Science has not been able to duplicate what nature has perfected over millions of years, and I don't believe we ever will.

Unfortunately, harmful chemical preservatives and other artificial additives are the norm in most pet foods. Some are intentionally added by the manufacturer, while others come from the herbicides, insecticides, and pesticides used by farmers to boost crop yields. Many pet foods advertised as "preservative-free" do, in fact, contain preservatives. As the law is currently written, manufacturers don't have to list preservatives that they themselves did not add. Many preservatives make their way into pet food at rendering plants before the meat is even sent to the manufacturer. An analysis of several pet foods labeled "chemical free" or "all natural ingredients" found synthetic antioxidants in all samples.[5] With continued use, low levels of these synthetic antioxidants may build up in the tissues; ingestion of small doses over time may be just as toxic as a single large dose. About 60 percent of all herbicides, 90 percent of all fungicides, and 30 percent of all insecticides are considered to be cancer causing in and of themselves. [6,7]

Two well-known carcinogens, butylated hydroxytoluene (BHT) and butylated hydroxyanisole (BHA), are used as preservatives in both animal and human food. These carcinogens were found in a variety of tests to induce double-strand DNA breaks, DNA adducts, mutations, and chromosomal aberrations.[8] Researchers have concluded that at some level of ingestion, synthetic antioxidants are inducers or promoters of neoplasia and that the true safety and toxic levels are not well known or adequately researched in dogs or cats.

Although you won't see it on the label, since it is often added at the rendering plant and not by the manufacturer, ethoxyquin (EQ) is used to preserve most dry pet food.[9] First used as a rubber stabilizer, EQ is the most powerful of all preservatives and may be the most toxic. Originally, it was permitted in livestock food. So since pet food is considered animal feed, the use of EQ is also permitted in pet food. The fish industry uses high levels of EQ; factory workers exposed to it exhibited side effects similar to those of agent orange: a dramatic rise in liver or kidney damage, cancerous skin lesions, hair loss, blindness, leukemia, fetal abnormalities, and chronic diarrhea. In animals, EQ has been linked to immune deficiency syndrome; spleen, stomach, and liver cancers; and a host of allergies.[10]

Many factors can lead to cancer. Impurities in water, food, and air; immunosuppressive drugs; and poor nutrition all play a major role. More research needs to be done to determine the safety levels of synthetic antioxidants and other chemicals found in food manufactured for our dogs and cats.

chapter 3

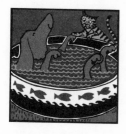

Real Vitamins for Health and Healing

VITAMINS ARE EXTREMELY COMPLEX ORGANIC SUBSTANCES needed in small amounts in the diet. They are essential for both human and animal metabolic processes. The body is not capable of producing sufficient quantities of vitamins to supply its needs under normal circumstances. There are some vitamin-like substances that are not considered essential since the body's tissues are usually able to produce them in sufficient amounts. Each vitamin has its own unique functions in the body and cannot be replaced by any other substance.

Real vitamins are too complex to develop in a test tube and put in a bottle—even with man's modern technological advances. What man has developed is a "vitamin fraction" or a small part of a real vitamin and given it a name such as ascorbic acid for vitamin C. As you will see, ascorbic acid is only a small part of vitamin C and physiologically does not act as "real" vitamin C. Real vitamins can only be obtained from foods or food concentrates and not from synthesized artificial vitamins. Vitamins are actually a group of chemically related compounds. Once a vitamin is separated or fractionated into a single compound, it no longer behaves as nature intended the vitamin to behave. Thus, synthesized vitamins have little or no value and may even be dangerous with prolonged use.

Extensive research is elucidating the various roles and interrelationships of vitamin compounds or complexes. Though the nature, chemical structure, and composition of most vitamins are known and many vitamin fractions have been isolated and synthesized (parts of vitamins produced in the laboratory), research has really only scratched the surface of identifying all the interdependent and interactive components of vitamin complexes.[1]

Each dog or cat is unique in its nutritional requirement. One dog may require five times as much vitamin A or vitamin D as another dog. I believe that there is biochemical individuality among animals and that nutritional needs differ quantitatively from animal to animal. Although all dogs require the same nutritional needs, each individual animal has a biochemical pattern all its own. This pattern is dependent upon circumstantial and environmental conditions.

With food and food concentrates containing whole nutritional complexes, the body can choose the nutrients it needs for assimilation and excrete what it does not need. With synthetic or fractionated vitamins, the body has no choice. It must handle the vitamin as a foreign substance or drug, and then toxicity or chemical imbalance may occur.

Though certain intestinal bacteria can produce vitamin B_{12}, vitamin K, and B-complex factors, with rare exceptions, nearly all vitamins in food are either directly or indirectly produced by plants. Vitamin-rich whole foods are still the only source of virtually all the vitamins. Some of the best sources include seeds, nuts, whole grains, eggs, vegetables, yeasts and yeast extracts, liver and other organ meats, and fruits. In humans, clinical vitamin deficiencies are rare in industrialized countries such as the United States. However, subclinical nutrient deficiencies are rampant and put a burden on our healthcare system. Signs of nutrient deficiencies may include bleeding gums, arthritis, stiff joints, easy bruising, dermatitis, any inflammatory disorders, cardiac problems, fatigue, gastrointestinal disorders, and dry skin. A subclinical deficiency means that the body's nutrient stores (vitamin, mineral, trace element) have been gradually drained, resulting in loss of optimal health and impairment of body processes leading to a variety of degenerative diseases.[2]

An important point is that there is no such thing as a 100 percent balanced diet for dogs and cats that is processed and bagged or canned. This is a sad myth perpetrated by big industry and uninformed professionals. One cannot substitute synthetic vitamins and "dead" processed food for raw, "live" natural foods. If one must feed dead processed foods due to convenience and time constraints, then one should supplement the diet with real "live" foods or food concentrates. (We will see in chapter 5, the diet section of this book, how easy this is to do.)

When foods are processed, their nutrients are destroyed and they become unwholesome. This is done to prolong shelf life. Wholesome foods in their natural unrefined state, the whole plant or animal, insofar as it is edible, contain all of the food elements conducive to good health. Nutritive deficits cannot be rectified by a synthetic vitamin pill consisting of chemically isolated vitamin fractions. Remember, we have only scratched the surface of knowledge when it comes to nutrition. There are many nutrients in nature yet to be discovered. The 100 percent complete processed food will never be enough for optimum health.

IN NATURE, VITAMINS COME IN COMPLEXES

In nature, vitamins appear in complexes and not as isolated chemicals. For example, if there is a shortage of one B-group vitamin, there will be a shortage of several other B-group vitamins. A synthetic vitamin pill cannot make up for all the shortages. The point is important because only whole foods contain all *related* nutrients (vitamins, minerals, trace elements, enzymes, coenzymes, amino acids, fatty acids, and unknown factors). These nutrients function together for the biochemical equilibrium of the body. Supplying single vitamins in supplements is dangerous and unwholesome and can lead to further depletions and imbalances.[3, 4]

As stated before, vitamins are too complex to be synthesized in a test tube. It took nature hundreds of millions of years to perfect these nutrients and for animals to adapt to them. A vitamin consists of not only the organic nutrients identified as the vitamin, but also enzymes, coenzymes, antioxidants, and trace element activation. Since enzymes are proteins, they must contain amino acids and trace elements. Dr. Royal Lee, a pioneer in nutrition research, says, "In fact, every mineral needed by the living cell is commonly found in a natural assemblage of vitamin concentrates."[5] These components are only effective when in the proper natural state.

The truth of the matter is that synthetic isolated vitamin supplements act more like drugs than natural vitamins. Supplements must be food concentrates, intact, integrated, with their vitamin complexes incorporated so as to retain their functional and nutritional integrity. They must contain all the factors indigenous to food—both known and unknown factors—in their entirety. Chemically pure vitamins when ingested must be put in the proper combination with the other natural components of that vitamin complex to be utilized by the body. This is potentially dangerous because introducing one component can use up the missing factors from the body's reserves and this can lead to a deficiency of other components. Therefore, since these synergistic factors are normally an integral part of the vitamin complex necessary to its fractional form, a deficiency of that vitamin itself may develop. In other words, taking a chemically pure crystalline form can lead to a vitamin deficiency of the very vitamin taken. Also, the body treats the synthetic as a drug and tries to rid it from the body quickly by funneling it through the kidneys and excreting it through the urine.[6]

Epidemiologic studies of nutrients in humans hold much public interest. Physicians and their patients are watching the current number of studies on antioxidants (fractions of vitamin complexes) such as beta carotene, ascorbic acid (fractionated vitamin C), and alpha-tocopheral (fractionated vitamin E) in the prevention of degenerative diseases. The results have been conflicting. However, the most important message is that chemically synthesized supplements are no substitute for real food complexes. Foods contain an intricate, interconnected network of components of known and unknown nutrients, which work together for the effectiveness or formation of the body. Chemically isolated and synthetic vitamins are devoid of all their synergists. The body treats natural and synthetic vitamins differently. When defining carbohydrates, vitamins, fats, or any other food element, each must be considered as a complex, made up of many forms, and the best philosophy is to get as many forms as possible.

Years ago, a Cuban study found that fish liver oil (vitamin A) had antihypertensive effects. However, when American doctors tried to duplicate the study, they failed. Later, it was discovered that the vitamin A concentrate used in the U.S. was refined and had eliminated key nutrients that affected high blood pressure. It is important to remember that a vitamin is a complex assembly of food catalysts, which must not be altered to retain its function.[7]

SYNTHETIC VITAMINS ARE FRACTIONS OF THE REAL THING

From a biochemical standpoint, synthetic vitamins are a mirror image of just a portion of the real, biologically active vitamin complex. They are as different as right- and left-hand gloves. They may appear identical but react in different ways. The body can tell the difference and treats synthetic vitamins as drugs and not as nutrients as the manufacturers would have you believe. (By the way, synthetic vitamins are produced by several pharmaceutical companies.) One must be careful when taking synthetic vitamins because high doses can be toxic. For example, high doses of ascorbic acid (synthetic vitamin C) can cause kidney stones, while high doses of kiwi fruit (a source of natural vitamin C) will not. Ingestion of high doses of synthetic vitamin A can be dangerous, while ingestion of natural vitamin A in the form of egg yolk, butter, or cod liver oil is safe. Synthetic vitamin A has had temporary positive results in severe vitamin A deficiency in children with measles; however, these are partial results, only masking the symptoms temporarily.[8]

THE B-COMPLEX:
THE DANGER OF ISOLATING VITAMINS

The B vitamins are found in nature together and not as isolated components. They always occur together in nature. Good sources of vitamin B-complex in food are Brewer's yeast, liver, whole grains (bran and germ), organ meats, nuts, beans, and peas. The B-complex vitamins have a wide range of functions in the body. All cells require this vitamin complex, which aids in the oxidation of carbohydrates, proteins, and foods; cell respiration; and cellular mineral and energy production. The B-complex is essential for the normal functioning of the nervous system, the maintenance of muscle tone, and the stimulation of digestive and insulin secretions. It is important to the health and normal function of the heart, liver, eyes, skin, hair, endocrine system (adrenal, thyroid, pituitary, ovaries, testis), spleen, thymus gland, pancreas, and kidneys. The B vitamins are also important for red blood cell production and the proper functioning of the immune system.[9]

In nature, there exists such a close interrelationship among the B vitamins that an inadequate intake of one may impair the utilization of others. Furthermore, large doses of one member of the complex can create a vitamin imbalance and precipitate deficiency of other members of the complex. Thus, the B-complex should be taken as a whole with all members (known and unknown) present, rather than any single substance or isolated substances of the group. In nature, the B-complex can be found in foods, but never does one find a single B vitamin isolated from the rest. Virtually all preparations of single B vitamins as well as combining many single B vitamins in one supplement ("high potency") are synthetic or at least chemically isolated unnatural forms.

Large doses of a single synthetic B vitamin have been shown to induce deficiencies of other B factors in humans. For instance, injections of B_1 (thiamine) results in symptoms of pellagra, known as a vitamin B_3 (niacin amide) deficiency in people.[10] Overloading with one component of the B-complex produces a definite deficiency of other components. The whole complex from "live" foods is needed for best results. Animals and humans should get their B-complex vitamins from several sources. There are still nutrients yet to be discovered in foods. These "unknown" nutrients have synergistic beneficial effects, which can only be obtained from different food factors.

A group of mice were placed on a synthetic diet that included all "necessary" nutrients. They grew for a few days and then became static in weight. After twenty to thirty days, the animals began to lose their hair and developed hunched backs. Another group of mice were placed on the same diet with whole yeast added. Once this "natural" food was introduced, none of the symptoms of the first group developed.[11] Benefits from synthetic vitamins are short-lived, and after a time, the benefits are reversed.

ASCORBIC ACID AND VITAMIN C ARE NOT THE SAME

Though dogs and cats can produce vitamin C under times of stress and disease, an addition to the diet will be beneficial. Though the established health community considers vitamin C and ascorbic acid as one in the same, nothing can be farther from the truth.

Ascorbic acid is present in natural vitamin C complex, but only serves as an antioxidant, preventing the deterioration of the functional important part of the complex. Vitamin C, as found in whole foods, contains rutin (vitamin P), the bioflavonoid complex, the K factor, the J factor, tyrosinase (an enzyme), ascorbic acid, ascorbigen, and unknown nutritional factors not yet discovered.[12]

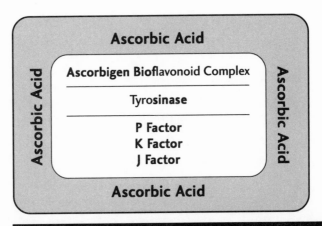

FIGURE 3.1 Vitamin C Complex

As you can see, ascorbic acid serves as a protector of the functional part of vitamin C. Rutin (P factor) is especially important in strengthening blood vessels and other collagen containing tissues. The K factor supports the clotting mechanism, and the J factor supports the oxygen carrying capacity of the blood. The bioflavonoids play a multitude of roles, and tyrosinase activates the vitamin. Tyrosinase is depended upon organic copper for its production. So, as you can see, the natural vitamin C complex is truly *complex*—in both its construction and its functions.

Natural vitamin C complex assists in a multitude of normal bodily functions. Major roles are in the formation of collagen, endothelial tissues (cells that line blood and lymph vessels), the heart, and other body cavities. It is important in wound healing, hormonal functions, bone growth and strength, glutathione concentration (an important antioxidant and cofactor for enzymes that helps against heart disease, cancer, and inflammation), anemia, metabolism of amino acids, hormone production and metabolism, pulmonary function, and mineral uptake and distribution. There is evidence that natural vitamin C—but not ascorbic acid—supports the immune system in preventing the development of cancer. White blood cells carry more vitamin C than any other cell in the body—which explains why it is important to ingest extra vitamin C containing foods during stress and disease.

> **Natural sources of vitamin C complex:** acerola berry, kiwi fruit, strawberries, citrus fruits, pineapple, guava, broccoli, kale, peppers (especially red), beets, spinach, collards, corn, parsley, turnip greens, raw milk, and adrenal glands.

Vitamins are required only in small amounts and have their most potent function when ingested as a whole food complex. All of the synergists are contained in the whole complex and work together to produce the greatest benefit. Potatoes, which contain only a small amount of vitamin C complex compared to citrus fruit, prevented scurvy in Northern Europe in the nineteenth century.[13] The so-called vitamin C fraction of ascorbic acid, even in large amounts, cannot cure scurvy; it functions more as a drug and not a nutrient.

Subclinical scurvy in dogs and cats may be more common than suspected. Signs may include dermatitis, intervertebral disc lesions, respiratory problems, arthritis, skin infections, gingivitis, poor wound healing, extreme weakness, muscle cramps, and weak ligaments.

According to a study from the USDA Agriculture Research Service, moderate vitamin C deficiency in humans results in a "compromised" immune system. Taking ascorbic acid does not provide the same protection as ingesting food sources of vitamin C complex. Daily intake of ascorbic acid supplements reduces the total white blood cell count, compromising the immune system rather than assisting it. When vitamin C complex is consumed in food form at 50mg or more per day, the white blood cell count remains normal. High dietary intake of vitamin C and the resulting healthy blood levels have been shown to protect against the development of chronic respiratory symptoms, while lower intakes are associated with significantly impaired pulmonary function. Ascorbic acid does not improve pulmonary or respiratory health.[14]

Inflammation is a natural process following tissue insult or injury. In the case of an upper respiratory infection caused by a change of temperature, pollution, virus, etc., inflammation appears in the mucous membrane linings of the nasal passages and/or sinuses. The body responds in several different ways: (1) releases enzymes to digest intracellular proteins of injured cells, releasing histamine and other chemicals; (2) increases blood flow to the area after the action exerted by histamine to isolate the injured area, which results in redness, heat (fever), and congestion; (3) increases white blood cell migration to the area (white blood cells phagocytize cellular debris, which becomes pus while increased mucous secretion makes up phlegm); and (4) organizes other while blood cells to repair tissue by laying the matrix for the rebuilding of damaged tissues.

Medications such as aspirin, steroids, antihistamines, and ascorbic acid interfere with the initial stages of inflammation. Thus, the symptoms of inflammation may lessen or disappear, but the natural healing process now sabotaged by these medical interventions cannot accomplish what nature intended. Fever may lessen, redness and congestion may abate, and mucous may dry up; however, the price paid may be a slow, healing process. Chicken soup with vegetables is nature's medicine and will do more for an upper respiratory infection than any antibiotic, antihistamine, or ascorbic acid can ever accomplish.

The rutin and bioflavonoid components of the vitamin C complex are important in stopping capillary hemorrhages, lowering high blood pressure, fibrin formation in blood clotting, and formation in intercellular substances for blood vessels.

Tyrosinase and organic copper as part of the vitamin C complex are essential to all muscles, especially the heart muscle, which undergoes atrophy with low tyrosinase levels. Increased vitamin C intake can greatly help heart associated problems. As thousands of milligrams of ascorbic acid are ingested, organic copper and tyrosinase are depleted from the body. These vital nutrients are needed by the body to make ATP (energy), collagen (glue that holds muscles and joints together), and melatonin. There are probably other functions that are jeopardized as well.

More than one hundred studies have found that people who eat diets rich in fresh fruits and vegetables are about half as likely to develop cancer as people who eat few fruits and vegetables. Of forty-six studies comparing healthy people to those with cancer, thirty-three found that cancer risk decreases when people get at least 60 mgs of vitamin C per day from food. A study at the Mayo Clinic gave 150 cancer patients either 10,000 mgs of ascorbic acid a day or a placebo. The ascorbic acid neither shrank tumors nor lengthened survival time any better than did the placebo.[15] Large doses of ascorbic acid have numerous adverse affects, including weakening of red blood cells leading to hemolysis or destruction of these cells, irritation of the mucous membranes lining of the gastrointestinal tract, renal calcification, and interference with Vitamin B_{12} and vitamin A metabolism. It has also been shown that high levels of ascorbic acid taken daily, depletes blood copper levels with serious ramifications. Both red blood cells and the liver cells can lose copper resulting in diminished superoxide dismutase (S.O.D.) and a consequential decrease in adrenal hormones (epinephrine and norepinephrine). As can be imagined, all body processes are affected. Organic copper is essential to the development of red blood cells, and any interference contributes to anemia.

The adrenal glands contain large quantities of vitamin C, which exceeds the concentration of all other tissues. Epinephrine, norepinephrine, corticosteroids, mineralcorticoids, and sex steroids (small amounts) are secreted by the adrenals. There is evidence to suggest that vitamin C is involved in the production of these hormones by the adrenal glands. Eskimos and Canadian Indians ate the adrenal glands of the animals they hunted to prevent scurvy. Ascorbic acid, on the other hand, inhibits the production of adrenal hormones. Dogs and cats given ascorbic acid may become prone to the formation of oxalate-type urinary bladder stones.

Chemically synthesized ascorbic acid does not function as natural vitamin C complex. Man cannot produce in a test tube what took nature millions of years to evolve. For optimum health, make sure your pet receives its vitamin C from food sources—not a convenient pill.

THE CONFUSION OVER VITAMIN E

Vitamin E was first identified in 1922. Since then much confusion and controversy has surrounded this all-important vitamin. It was demonstrated that a diet deficient in certain lipids resulted in reproductive failure in rats. The missing substance turned out to be vitamin E.

Many professionals use the terms tocopherol and tocotrienol as "vitamin E," but this is simplifying the case. There is much more to the vitamin E complex. There are at least eight forms of tocopherol in food (alpha, beta, eta, gamma, delta, epsilon, zeta, etc.), which serve as antioxidants to protect the other important and potent components of the vitamin E complex from immediate oxidation or destruction.[16]

Vitamin E complex is important in stabilizing cell membranes; protecting cells and tissues such as lungs, skin, eyes, liver, muscles, kidneys, and heart from free radical damage and damage from pollutants; helping to regulate the use and storage of vitamin A; protecting red blood cells from damage; and preventing cancer.

Vitamin E in foods, once separated from its whole complex, is not stable when stored. To improve its stability or shelf life and thus make it commercially viable, drug companies esterify it, a chemical conversion to protect the vitamin from deterioration. In nature, all foods are designed to deteriorate or break down once they are damaged, a way of recycling the components back to nature. Stabilizing a vitamin fraction or esterifying it alters the vitamin so that it is no longer a food component and/or cannot be properly used by the body as an isolated food factor. Manufacturers refine out the whole complex, leaving only one tiny portion, which does not deteriorate as a natural food does; it is only a dead chemical remnant. While esterification makes alpha-tocopherol "stable" against oxidation—giving it a long shelf life—it also makes alpha-tocopherol ineffective as an antioxidant; in other words, thanks to processing, it is no longer able to react with oxygen.

Biochemists are simply unable to duplicate nature's beauty and wisdom. Even the so-called "mixed togopherol" contains a set amount of esterified d-alpha-tocopherol and lesser amounts of a few other tocopherols and/or tocotrienols. Only the rarely found vitamin E complex supplement contains the whole complex. This complex contains oil extracted from grains or dehydrated vegetables (whole pea plants and alfalfa) that are minimally processed to remove only the water by freeze drying. This type of food concentrate contains all the natural factors associated with and part of the vitamin complex, including unsaturated fatty acids; vitamin A, D, and K complexes; and trace elements such as selenium, zinc, manganese, enzymes, etc.[17] It has now been established that there are interactions between vitamin E and other nutrients in foods. Recognized but then forgotten was the fact that whole natural vitamin E, such as found in wheat germ, beans, or other foods, loses up to 90 percent of its potency when separated from its natural synergists. These synergists are lost in the distillation process to separate the alpha-tocopherol from the rest of the food. The vitamin E complex is surrounded by the protective antioxidant tocopherols and includes vitamin E_2, vitamin E_3, unsaturated fatty acids (F_1 and F_2) xanthine, lipositols, selenium, coenzymes, and more known and unknown components.[18]

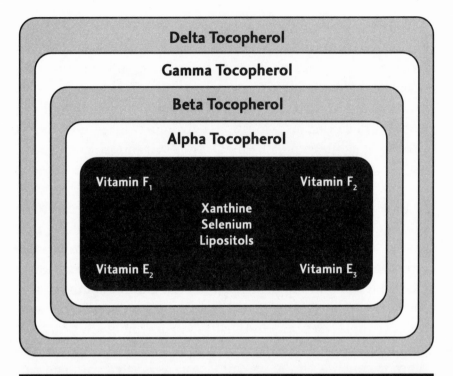

FIGURE 3.2 Vitamin E Complex

As you can see in figure 3.2, the vitamin E complex is a lot more than alpha-tocopherol, the so-called vitamin E in supplements. It is interesting how nutrients in nature interact with each other. As if by design, there appears to be a relationship between the concentration of linoleic acid in various plant oils and the concentration of tocopherols. The potent antioxidant effects of the tocopherol prevent its oxidation of the relatively unstable fatty acids. Tocopherols protect the linoleic acid and other oil constituents making up the vitamin E complex.

Traditionally, vitamin E complex has been thought of as the reproductive vitamin; however, it is also necessary for proper functioning of the central nervous system; maintenance of all muscles (especially the heart); cancer prevention; intracellular respiration; glandular functions (thyroid, adrenal); healthy skin and hair; red blood cell and blood vessel integrity; liver, kidney, and lung integrity; and detoxification, just to name a few.[19]

In nature, there is an interrelationship between various vitamins and minerals, and they all play a synergistic role with one another for optimum health. For example, selenium always appears with vitamin E complex in foods and functions as an activator of the complex. There are other important nutrients that cooperate with vitamin E complex; they include vitamins A, C, K, B_6, and $B_{12;}$ folic acid; pantothenic acid; zinc; iron; and essential fatty acids. This is another good reason to get your nutrients from foods or food concentrates and not from fractionated vitamin pills.

One study found purified alpha-tocopherol was of no value in the treatment of muscular weakness due to vitamin E deficiency, while wheat germ oil, a source of whole vitamin E complex, successfully treated the weakness.[20]

It has been demonstrated in humans that low concentrations of vitamin E in blood plasma pose a greater risk for dying from heart disease than elevated cholesterol levels or even hypertension.[21] In the 1950s, Dr. W.E. Shute gave 8,600 cardiovascular patients wheat germ oil, which contains the whole vitamin E complex. He found a 42 to 53 percent improvement in overall cardiovascular health.[22] Such studies provide a good reason to supplement a heart patient with wheat germ. I personally eat eggs, which are extremely high in vitamin E, several times a week. Both dogs and cats enjoy raw eggs, and they are good for them. I prefer eggs from free-range fed chickens. Some farms are now feeding chickens flax seeds, which is high in omega-3 fatty acids. This is also excellent for cardiovascular and neurologic health. Pure alpha-tocopherol is in reality a drug and not a nutrient, as most people believe. As you know, any drug can have side effects. Large doses of alpha-tocopherol have been shown to cause nausea, flatulence, diarrhea, and bone decalcification.[23] Megadoses have been shown to cause a decrease in thyroid hormone, growth retardation, reduced red blood cells or anemia, and muscle weakness in test animals.[24]

Vitamin E is the major chain-breaking antioxidant in body tissue and is considered the first line of defense against lipid perioxidation, which protects all membranes at an early stage of free radical through its free radical-involving activity. Antioxidant defenses that protect the body from free radical damage include the enzymes superoxide dismutate, catalase, and glutathione peroxides; vitamins C and E; carotenoids; alpha-lipoic acid; and the bioflavanoids. There is extensive evidence to implicate free radicals in the development of degenerative disease and conditions.[25]

Both exogenous and hereditary factors are believed to be involved in cancer development. In humans, it has been estimated that 80 to 90 percent of all cancers are environmentally induced, approximately 35 percent of them by diet.[26] Research data have shown that free radicals frequently have a role in the process of cancer initiation and promotion. Results of cell and animal studies suggest that vitamin E and the other antioxidants alter cancer incidence and growth through their actions as anti-carcinogens, quenching free radicals or reacting with cancer cell by-products.[27]

It has been estimated that approximately 40 percent of the factors influencing life expectancy can be controlled, which suggests not only that length of life can be extended, but also quality of life can be enhanced through better health. An important area of research on aging suggests that free radical damage to body cells leads to the pathological changes associated with aging.[28, 29]

It has been suggested that free radical generation associated with aging may be a contributory factor in the depressed immune response documented in aged rodents and that improved antioxidant status may have an immuno-stimulatory effect.[30]

Increasing research evidence implicates free radical mediated cell damage in the development of various degenerative diseases and conditions. The body's susceptibility to free radical stress and peroxidative damage is related to the balance between free radical load and the adequacy of antioxidant defenses. The majority of studies in both humans and animals have shown that increased intake of vitamin E is associated with decreased risk of degenerative diseases. As research continues on the beneficial effects of vitamin E and the other antioxidants in counteracting oxidative damage in the body, it would appear prudent to increase intakes of food high in vitamin E and other antioxidant nutrients to provide protection from the increasingly high free radical levels present in the environment.

Natural vitamin E is at least ten times as biologically active as the synthetic form.[31] The isolated alpha-tocopherol in high doses reverses any beneficial physiological effects and produces the same symptoms as a deficiency. Vitamin E is a complex of nutritional factors and not just alpha-tocopherol or mixed tocopherols alone. Other important workers in the vitamin E complex are xanthine (spares up to 50 percent of tocopherol requirement), lipositols (help cholesterol metabolism and steroid hormone processes), vitamin E_2 and vitamin F_2 (aid assimilation of blood reserves of fats and proteins), vitamin F_1 (unsaturated fatty acid factor important to cellular differentiation and calcium assimilation) discovered in wheat germ oil, and even more unknown factors yet to be discovered.[32] There is just no substitute for a good, wholesome, raw organic food diet. Taking shortcuts by substituting so-called vitamin pills for good nutrition will harm both humans and their animal companions. You can prevent many diseases by taking a little time to feed good food to your dog or cat. Only foods contain real vitamin E complex.

> **Natural sources of vitamin E:** Sources of vitamin E are seeds, nuts, whole grains, raw eggs, raw milk, and green leafy vegetables. Interestingly, raw milk contains vitamins A, B-complex, C, D, and E; conjugated linoleic acid; essential fatty acids; all amino acids (some destroyed by pasteurization); precursors for glutathion synthesis (most important antioxidant); more than thirty enzymes; many trace elements and minerals; and as yet undiscovered nutrients. As you can see, raw milk is nearly a perfect food. It is a shame that man has taken a gift from nature and ruined it by pasteurization. Perhaps one day man will see the error in his ways.

A GUIDE TO NATURAL VITAMINS

One way to ensure that your pet is eating nutritious food is to be aware of the vitamins in your pet's food. What vitamins are important for the health and well-being of your dog or cat? And what are natural sources of these vitamins?

Vitamin A and Carotenoids

Vitamin A plays an important role in the health of both dogs and cats. Carotenoids, however, are important only to dogs. Cats lack an essential enzyme necessary to convert beta carotene into vitamin A.[33] Sources of vitamin A are found in animal tissues and vegetables, while carotenes are found only in vegetation. This is one more good reason why cats are strict carnivores, while dogs may be considered omnivores. Minimum requirements for vitamin A are 500 IU/KG per daily ration (IU is international units).

Vitamin A performs several chores: It is essential in the prevention of xeropathalmia, which is a drying and thickening condition of the conjunctiva of the eye. It also helps maintain the integrity of the epithelial and mucosal surfaces and their secretions. The mucosal surfaces are the first line of defense against infections.

The immune system is also quite dependent on vitamin A. A deficiency of vitamin A can result in atrophy of lymph glands, decreased number of lymphocytes, and a reduced B- and T cell function.[34] Children given vaccines and vitamin A showed a much greater antibody response than vitamin A deficient children.[35] Normal T cell counts were restored with vitamin A administration. Not only does vitamin A increase the number of T cells, but it also appears to enable T cells to respond to pathogens. Severe vitamin A deficiency also leads to atrophy of the thymus and spleen and a dramatic decrease in the number of white blood cells.[36] High levels of vitamin A administration have been shown to stimulate and/or enhance numerous immune processes, including inducing the activity of cell-mediated immunity that destroys cancer cells, natural killer cell activity, lymphocyte production, phagocytes, and antibody production. Furthermore, vitamin A has also been shown to promote the growth of the thymus gland.[37] I prefer vitamin A from food sources only.

> **Natural sources of vitamin A:** Some of the highest concentrations of vitamin A are found in the livers of beef, calf, and chickens. Vitamin A also can be found in eggs, butter, raw milk, and cod liver oil.

Carotenoids

This subject matter is strictly applicable to dogs and not cats. As previously stated, cats lack a crucial enzyme needed to convert beta carotene into vitamin A.

Carotenoids are naturally occurring colorful compounds that are abundant as pigments in plants. Although more than six hundred specific carotenoids have been identified, only a limited number are important. The major ones are alpha-carotene, beta carotene, lutein, zeaxanthin, cryptoxanthin, and lycopene.[38, 39]

A number of carotenoids are effective in preventing or controlling free radical generation. These carotenoids can work together or with other antioxidants to prevent the generation of free radicals. Other antioxidant defenses include vitamins C and E, alpha lipoic acid, polyphenols, and the enzymes superoxide dismutase, catalase, and glutathione peroxidase. Each antioxidant is important, and each has a separate role in protection against free radical damage.[40] Oxidative damage resulting from free radical attack has been linked to the onset of a number of degenerative diseases and conditions.[41] Many research studies show that carotenoids play a role in preventing or minimizing free radical damage associated with cancer, coronary heart disease, cataracts, and age-related macular degeneration. Though these studies are with human subjects, one may extrapolate for canine patients.

Despite their similarities in structure, carotenoids have diverse biological functions. Certain carotenoids are precursors to vitamin A and can be metabolically converted (except in cats) into vitamin A in the body. Beta carotene has the highest potential vitamin A activity; other provitamin A carotenoids include alpha-carotene and cryptoxanthin.

As mentioned previously, carotenoids are effective quenchers of singlet oxygen (free radicals). Lycopene exhibits the highest free radical quenching activity.[42]

Boosting the Immune System

Carotenoids have demonstrated a number of immune-enhancing effects in recent studies.[43] Originally, researchers thought that the immune-enhancing effects of carotenes were because of their conversion to vitamin A. They now know that carotenes exert many immune-enhancing effects independent of any vitamin A activity.

One of the most interesting studies was done on healthy human volunteers. This study showed that beta carotene significantly increased Helper T-4 lymphocytes by 30 percent in seven days and all T cells after fourteen days.[44] T-4 lymphocytes play a critical role in determining host immune status. This study indicates that oral beta carotene may be effective in increasing the immunological competence of a patient who has a depressed T-Helper lymphocyte count such as in cancer or viral infections. Since the thymus gland is so susceptible to free radical damage, beta carotene may be even more helpful in protecting the immune system than vitamin A. I recommend only natural beta carotene from food or food concentrates.

Numerous studies have demonstrated that people with the highest intake of carotenoid-rich fruits and vegetables and/or high blood levels of specific carotenoids usually have the lowest risk of certain types of cancer. In one study, serum concentrations of total carotenoids, cryptoxanthin, and alpha-carotene were lower in cancer patients than in controls.[45] In another study, increased dietary beta carotene consumption was associated with a lower risk for endometrial cancer.[46] In other studies, dietary beta carotene consumption was associated with reduced lung cancer risk and serum total carotenoid and beta carotene concentrations were lower in lung cancer patients.[47, 48]

British researchers may have discovered a possible mechanism by which the immune system fights cancer and infections. To identify and destroy cancer cells, white blood cells called monocytes have to first distinguish the cancer cells from normal cells. A protein called MHC II, which sits on the surface of monocytes, in a sense, searches for cancer cells.[49] When the MHC II protein notices a cancer cell, the monocytes attract the attention of other immune system cells, which move in and attack the cancer cell. If monocytes don't have MHC II proteins, which are akin to a biological sensor, the cancer may go unnoticed and grow. This may be one way in which the immune system is involved in tumor surveillance. This may also be a good way to help fight off infectious diseases.

Natural sources of carotenoids: The richest dietary sources of carotenoids are fruits and vegetables, apricots, cantaloupe, carrots, leafy green vegetables, pumpkin, sweet potato, winter squash, tomatoes, red peppers, mangoes, broccoli, kale, and Swiss chard.[50] There are other sources but this covers the bulk of them. Based on current research data, increased intake of a mixture of natural carotenoids, rather than beta carotene alone, may be a greater benefit in disease prevention and treatment.

Vitamin D

The term vitamin D covers a number of related compounds that have activity associated with vitamin D. The two most important are vitamin D_2 (ergocalciferol) and D_3 (cholecarciferol). Biochemical conversion of vitamin D occurs in the liver, kidney, and skin to produce physiologically active forms of the vitamin. It is best known for its ability to stimulate the absorption of calcium.

Most mammals can form vitamin D_3 in the skin after exposure to ultraviolet light, and so do not require additional dietary supplement of the vitamin. For dogs and cats, the estimated dietary requirement of vitamin D is 50 I.U./Kg daily.

The most interesting fact about vitamin D_3 is that it acts more like a hormone than a vitamin. It not only regulates calcium homeostasis through hormonal-like action, but it regulates cellular differentiation and proliferation. Vitamin D_3's ability to regulate cells makes it an important tool in the prevention and controlling of cancer. Along with vitamin A, it works synergistically to induce certain cancer cells to differentiate into normal cells and to inhibit cancer cell proliferation. Among the cancers that vitamin D_3 has been shown to be effective against in humans are colorectal, breast, prostate, ovarian, leukemia, and lymphoma.[51, 52, 53]

> **Natural sources of vitamin D:** There are many sources of vitamin D, such as raw milk, cod liver oil, coldwater fish, egg yolk, and dark green leafy vegetables.

Thiamine (B₁)

Thiamine is converted in the liver, where it acts as a key coenzyme in carbohydrate metabolism. Thiamine deficiency will result in impairment of carbohydrate metabolism and accumulation of pyruvic and lactic acids within the body, leading to neurological signs in dogs and cats. Raw fish may contain thiaminase and produce a deficiency. Cooking and processing of foods readily destroys this vitamin, and so commercial food must be supplemental with vitamin B₁.

> **Natural sources of thiamine:** Thiamine is widely distributed in Brewer's yeast, whole cereal grains, egg yolk, various nuts, raw milk, and raw meat.[54] Daily requirements are 1.0 mg/kg for dogs and 3.0 mg/kg for cats.

Riboflavin (B₂)

Riboflavin is a constituent to a number of enzyme systems. Flavin-mononucleotide (FMN) and Flavin-adenine-dinucleotide (FAD), the coenzyme forms of this vitamin, are necessary for a number of enzyme systems and are needed in every living cell of the body. A deficiency of this vitamin in animals is probably rare. Riboflavin helps produce energy and regenerate glutathione, one of the main cellular protectors against free radical damage.[55] Animals with low levels of glutathione are prone to cataract formation, scaly skin, muscular weakness, anemia, and death.[56, 57]

> **Natural sources of B$_2$:** Rich sources of B$_2$ are organ meats (liver, kidney, heart), whole grains, raw milk, mushrooms, Brewer's yeast, and green leafy vegetables.[58]

Niacin (B$_3$)

Niacin includes either niacin (nicotinic acid or nicotinate) or niacinamide (nicotinamide).

Niacin is essential in the production of energy. It plays a role in the regulation of blood sugar, antioxidant mechanisms, and detoxification reactions. In addition to its nutritional effects, niacin exerts a favorable effect on several health conditions, especially high cholesterol levels.[59] In dogs, tryptophan is converted to niacin, which may lessen the requirements.

> **Natural sources of B$_3$:** Main food sources include liver and other organ meats, eggs, fish, legumes, whole grains, raw milk, and yeast.

Pyridoxine (B$_6$)

Pyridoxine (B$_6$) is an extremely important B vitamin, which is converted in the animal body to the active coenzyme pyridoxal phosphate. This coenzyme is involved in the formation of body proteins and structural compound chemical transmitters in the nervous system, red blood cells, and prostaglandins.

In humans, supplementation has been used in such conditions as asthma, cardiovascular disease, diabetes, epilepsy, and calcium oxalate stone formation.[60, 61] Pyridoxine daily requirements are 1.0 mg/kg for dogs and 4.0 mg/kg for cats. A B$_6$ deficiency in cats may manifest itself with irreversible kidney failure and calcium oxalate crystals.

Natural sources of B$_6$: Good sources include yeast, muscle meats, cereal grains, and vegetables.[62]

Biotin

Biotin is a B vitamin that functions in the manufacture and utilization of fats, carbohydrates, and certain amino acids. Since biotin is manufactured in the intestines by gut bacteria, a deficiency is unlikely. However, prolonged use of antibiotics may increase the likelihood of deficiency. A biotin deficiency may be characterized as dry, scaly skin; nausea; anorexia; and seborrhea.[63]

Pantothenic Acid (B$_5$)

Pantothenic acid, or vitamin B$_5$, is utilized in the manufacture of coenzyme A (CoA) and, thus, is involved in the metabolism of carbohydrates, fats, and some amino acids. A natural occurring deficiency is unlikely, since it is widely distributed in foods.

Folic Acid

Folic acid functions with B$_{12}$ in many body processes. It is critical in cellular division because it is necessary in DNA synthesis. It is also synthesized by intestinal bacteria.

In a folic acid deficiency, all cells are affected, especially the rapidly dividing cells such as red blood cells.[64] In pregnant humans, it is well known that a deficiency causes neural tube defects in babies.[65]

Natural sources of folic acid: Folic acid is widely distributed in foods such as Brewer's yeast, beef liver, rice, wheat bran, various beans, broccoli, and root vegetables.

Choline

Choline is essential in the manufacture of the important neu-rotransmitter acetylcholine and main components of our cell membranes, such as phosphatidyl choline (lecithin) and sphingo-myelin. It is also required for the proper metabolism of fats, pre-venting abnormal accumulation of fat in the liver. Because of choline's wide distribution in foods, a deficiency is unlikely; how-ever, the most likely related symptoms would involve fatty infil-tration of the liver and other signs of liver dysfunction.[66] Choline also increases acetylcholine content in the brain, which has been shown to improve memory.[67, 68]

> **Natural sources of choline:** Choline is found in grains; legumes; egg yolks; vegetables, such as cauliflower; whole grains; and liver.

Cobalamin (Vitamin B$_{12}$)

Vitamin B$_{12}$ is a general label for a group of essential biological compounds known as cobalamin. These are structurally related to hemoglobin in the blood; a deficiency of vitamin B$_{12}$ can cause anemia. The primary concern of conventional doctors is to main-tain adequate cobalamin status to prevent anemia. The most com-mon form of supplemented vitamin B$_{12}$ is called cyanocobalamin. However, vitamin B$_{12}$ is active in only two forms: methyl cobal-amin and adenosylcobalamin. Methyl cobalamin is active imme-diately upon absorption; cyanocobalamin must be converted by the liver to methyl cobalamin by removing the cyanide molecule and adding a methyl group.[69] Clinical trials have produced better results with methyl cobalamin than cyanocobalamin. However, in nature all of the B vitamins are found as a complex together.

Signs of vitamin B$_{12}$ deficiency may manifest themselves as anemia and neurologic deficits.[70] In persons over age sixty-five, it was found that as high as 42 percent may have a B$_{12}$ deficiency. In human patients, many neurological disorders have been treated with methylcobalamin. Published studies show that high doses of methylcobalamin are needed to regenerate neurons as well as the myelin sheath that protects axons and peripheral nerves. Let's look at a few human neurological diseases that are helped with methylcobalamin.

Bell's Palsy is a nonlethal paralysis of the facial nerve. Any or all branches of the nerve may be affected, and, in fact, victims may not be able to open an eye or close one side of the mouth. In one study, sixty patients were divided into three groups. One group was given steroids, one group was given steroids plus methylcobalamin, and the last group was given methylcobalamin by itself. The group on steroids only took 7.79 weeks to recover completely. The group on steroids plus methylcobalamin recovered in just 5.1 days.[71] We can certainly use methylcobalamin in geriatric vestibular syndrome, a commonly seen condition where elderly dogs have a head tilt and may circle to one side or another and appear disoriented. I have used an injectable form with good results along with acupuncture.

Diabetic neuropathy in humans has been shown to be helped after four months of oral administration of methylcobalamin. There were subjective improvements in burning sensations, numbness, loss of sensation, muscle cramps, reflexes, lower motor neuron weakness, and sensitivity to pain.[72]

Alzheimer's disease patients have significantly low levels of vitamin B_{12}. Marked mental improvements were noted in several studies when patients were supplemented with methylcobalamin.[73, 74, 75]

Mutiple sclerosis (MS) has a poor prognosis and features a widespread demyelination in the central nervous system. The coexistence of a vitamin B_{12} deficiency in MS may aggravate the disease or promote another cause of progressive demyelination.[76] Can methylcobalamin help degenerative myelopathy in German shepherds? I would like to see research on this devastating disease.

Natural sources of vitamin B$_{12}$: Foods that are found to have significant quantities of vitamin B$_{12}$ are liver, kidneys, clams, oysters, and sardines. Although intestinal bacteria also produce vitamin B$_{12,}$ vegetarian diets would be detrimental to both dogs and cats.

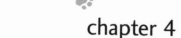

chapter 4

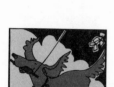

How the Decline in Minerals Affects Your Pet's Food

PRESIDENT FRANKLIN D. ROOSEVELT'S OBSERVATION IN 1937 regarding the importance of soil and health was prophetic. In a letter to the nation's governors, the president wrote: "A nation that destroys its soil destroys itself." Degenerative diseases started skyrocketing around this time and have been increasing ever since. I believe that the root of most diseases today in people and animals is due to nutrient depletion. Roosevelt's warning came during the aftermath of the Dust Bowl when soil erosion in numerous states resulted in large-scale crop and farm loss and rendered thousands of farms unemployed. As a result, the federal government established the Soil Conservation Service, which worked with individual states to correct the problem. By most accounts, the corrective measures of crop rotation, tree planting, contour plowing, and reserving lands for pastures have not worked. In fact, the advent of chemical fertilizers and pesticides has only made the matter worse.

Fewer than twenty-two years after Roosevelt's warning, the federal government reported that "the soil washed out of the fields of the United States each year would load a modern freight train long enough to reach around the world eighteen times." In 1984, conservative estimates placed topsoil loss in the U.S. at 1.7 billion tons a year. Today, that figure has increased to 3 billion. Worldwide, the estimate is 25.4 billion.

Most people probably have a hard time translating this ongoing problem into relevance in their own lives, but scientists, nutritionists, and doctors worldwide are beginning to view the degradation of the soil as a major health hazard because the soils have been depleted of nutrients. In fact, numerous studies are now suggesting that these nutrient-depleted soils are contributing to the major degenerative diseases of our time, including heart disease, cancer, and arthritis. Because the soils have been depleted of the minerals and trace elements that are necessary for optimal health, the food crops humans and animals eat from these soils are failing to supply us with the nutrients we need to ward off diseases.

So where did all the minerals go in the last one hundred years? In a stable ecosystem, minerals are drawn from the soil to the plants as they grow and bear fruit. When the plant dies, the minerals return to the earth for other plants to use. However, if the farmer hauls away the plants or their fruits and grains with a harvest, the minerals in them are removed from the cycle. The soil then becomes gradually depleted of its minerals, unless more are added to it in the form of fertilizer. Most soils will support only about ten years of intensive farming before the land becomes so mineral-depleted that it will no larger produce healthy plants.

In our high-tech world in which startling advances are made in both conventional and alternative medicine, we tend to forget that achieving optimal health can be as simple as providing the body with proper nutrition. Even when we do not forget, achieving that nutritional goal can be almost impossible because the very world in which we live bombards us with toxins on a daily basis.

We also have been lulled into a false sense of security by "popping" vitamins/mineral supplements. It is important to remember and emphasize that man cannot duplicate in a bottle of vitamins what nature has perfected within the plants for millions of years. The body treats artificial vitamins in tablet form, which are only parts of their natural vitamin complex, differently than natural vitamins obtained from foods. Whenever and wherever possible, I recommend eating fresh raw organic foods.

FERTILIZERS MAKE PLANTS LOOK NUTRITIOUS, BUT ARE THEY?

Modern farming practices over the last thirty years have greatly depleted our soils of vital nutrients. Today, artificial fertilizers containing nitrogen phosphorus and potassium (NPK) have largely replaced organic plants and animal parts in our soils. This disrupts the natural balance and cycle of plant—and ultimately animal and human—life on the planet.

There is a complex interaction between nutrients and soil organisms. The deficiency of a few nutrients (for example, sulfur and iron) will cause discoloration of plants, affecting their marketability.[1] Other elements are less crucial to productivity or appearance; however, they are extremely important to the nutritional value of the plants to animals and humans. If the secondary nutrients or trace elements become so depleted that it affects the productivity or appearance of a crop, these nutrients may be added to the soil. Iron is often added to fertilizers for commercial potato crops, which rapidly deplete the soil of the iron essential to the growth and appearance of the potato. Once again, the natural balance is disrupted.

The effects of chemical fertilizers are more complex than simple mineral loss. The addition of chemical nitrogen depletes both the vitamin C and the iron content of plants that grow from the fertilized soil.[2, 3] In addition, the potassium in NPK fertilizer is added in the form of potassium chloride, which means a ton of chloride is added along with every ton of potassium. The high levels of potassium inhibit plant absorption of magnesium.[4] Chloride leaches the soil of magnesium, zinc, and calcium.[5] Potassium chloride also alters the mineral balance so that selenium becomes bound in the soil and cannot be absorbed by plants.

The assault of decades of farming with NPK fertilizer has resulted in plants that look the same as they did generations ago, but which are depleted of the secondary plant nutrients and trace elements. Although the yield is adequate for commercial purposes, those plants are diseased. Like humans and animals, plants can suffer from mineral deficiency symptoms, which affect their immune systems. They are more prone to mold, fungus, and insect infestation, and they require large quantities of pesticides to keep them alive until they reach markets.

We now know that soil microorganisms are a key link in the mineralization of soil. Soil microbes ingest minerals from rocks in the soil; they also break down the organic matter of dead plants, releasing their minerals for use by other plants. Healthy soil is made up of bacteria, fungi, protozoa, nematodes, and micro arthropods. Minerals ingested by fungi and bacteria may not be available to plants, but the tiny predatory protozoa, nematodes, and micro arthropods eat bacteria, fungi, and each other and then release their nutrients in fecal matter.[6]

Unfortunately, chemical fertilizers and pesticides kill many of these beneficial organisms by providing unbalanced nutrient supply. The fertilizers can produce large yields for a while, but they eventually ruin the soil by disrupting the balance of the microorganisms, thus killing them off. The bacteria and fungi hold the soil together, so once they are greatly depleted or gone, soil erosion starts and carries nutrients away.[7] Pesticides affect the soil in much the same way that overuse of antibiotics affects humans and animals. At first, pesticides seem like a cure-all, but it soon becomes apparent that resistant organisms are beating the chemical warfare. The nutrient content of fruits, vegetables, grains, and meats have changed dramatically in the past thirty years. Table 4.1 shows changes in oranges, apples, and bananas.

TABLE 4.1

Changes in Mineral and Vitamin Content of Fruits 1963–1992 (per 100 grams)

ORANGES	1963	1992
Calcium	41 mg	40 mg
Iron	0.4 mg	0.1 mg
Magnesium	11 mg	10 mg
Phosphorus	20 mg	14 mg
Potassium	200 mg	181 mg
Vitamin A	200 I.U.	21 I.U.
Vitamin C	50 mg	53 mg
APPLES	**1963**	**1992**
Calcium	7 mg	7 mg
Iron	0.3 mg	0.18 mg
Magnesium	8 mg	5 mg
Phosphorus	10 mg	7 mg
Potassium	110 mg	115 mg
Vitamin A	90 I.U.	53 I.U.
Vitamin C	4 mg	5.7 mg
BANANAS	**1963**	**1992**
Calcium	8 mg	6 mg
Iron	0.7 mg	0.31 mg
Magnesium	33 mg	29 mg
Phosphorus	26 mg	20 mg
Potassium	370 mg	396 mg
Vitamin A	190 I.U.	87 I.U.
Vitamin C	10 mg	9.1 mg

Source: USDA, 1963[8] and 1997.[9]

The vitamin content of fruits and vegetables varies widely within a season depending on when they are picked. Vitamins are also less susceptible to depletion than minerals because the plant can make its own vitamins, while it must take minerals from the soil. According to table 4.1, vitamin A and iron have been the most depleted in the past thirty years. Table 4.2 shows mineral changes in various vegetables over a thirty-year period. Leafy green vegetables are promoted in many nutrition books as a good source of calcium, but depending on growth conditions, that may or may not be the case. Buy organically grown fruits and vegetables for higher nutritional content.

Table 4.2

**Changes in the Mineral Content of Vegetables
1963–1992 (per 100 grams)**

CARROT	1963	1992
Calcium	37 mg	27 mg
Iron	0.7 mg	0.5 mg
Magnesium	23 mg	15 mg
Phosphorus	36 mg	44 mg
Potassium	341 mg	323 mg
POTATOES	**1963**	**1992**
Calcium	7 mg	7 mg
Iron	0.6 mg	0.76 mg
Magnesium	34 mg	21 mg
Phosphorus	53 mg	46 mg
Potassium	407 mg	543 mg
CORN	**1963**	**1992**
Calcium	3 mg	3 mg
Iron	0.7 mg	0.52 mg
Magnesium	48 mg	37 mg
Phosphorus	111 mg	89 mg
Potassium	280 mg	270 mg
TOMATOES	**1963**	**1992**
Calcium	13 mg	5 mg
Iron	0.5 mg	0.45 mg
Magnesium	14 mg	11 mg
Phosphorus	27 mg	24 mg
Potassium	244 mg	222 mg

Table 4.2

Changes in the Mineral Content of Vegetables 1963–1992 (per 100 grams)

CELERY	1963	1992
Calcium	39 mg	40 mg
Iron	0.3 mg	0.4 mg
Magnesium	22 mg	11 mg
Phosphorus	28 mg	25 mg
Potassium	341 mg	287 mg
BROCCOLI	**1963**	**1992**
Calcium	103 mg	48 mg
Iron	1.10 mg	0.88 mg
Magnesium	24 mg	25 mg
Phosphorus	78 mg	66 mg
Potassium	382 mg	325 mg
ROMAINE LETTUCE	**1963**	**1992**
Calcium	68 mg	36 mg
Iron	1.4 mg	1.1 mg
Magnesium	n/a	6 mg
Phosphorus	25 mg	45 mg
Potassium	264 mg	290 mg
COLLARD GREENS	**1963**	**1992**
Calcium	203 mg	29 mg
Iron	1.00 mg	0.19 mg
Magnesium	57 mg	9 mg
Phosphorus	63 mg	10 mg
Potassium	401 mg	169 mg
SWISS CHARD	**1963**	**1992**
Calcium	88 mg	51 mg
Iron	3.2 mg	1.8 mg
Magnesium	65 mg	81 mg
Phosphorus	39 mg	46 mg
Potassium	550 mg	379 mg

Source: USDA, 1963[10] and 1997.[11]

Beef and chicken are the two most frequently consumed meats in the United States. There have been some nutritional declines in beef and chicken though not as dramatic as in plants. The most striking nutrient decline is that of vitamin A, which disappeared completely from beef and declined dramatically in chicken. Thiamine, one of the B vitamins, declined by 42 percent. Of the minerals, iron declined the most at an average of 28 percent. For many years, beef has been recommended for its iron contents; that advice no longer seems adequate.

Table 4.3

Changes in Nutrient Content of Beef and Chicken 1963–1992 (per 100 grams)

BEEF	1963	1992
Calcium	10 mg	8 mg
Iron	2.70 mg	1.73 mg
Magnesium	17 mg	16 mg
Phosphorus	156 mg	130 mg
Potassium	236 mg	228 mg
Vitamin A	40 I.U.	0
Thiamine	0.080 mg	0.038 mg
Riboflavin	0.160 mg	0.151 mg
Niacin	4.30 mg	4.48 mg
CHICKEN	**1963**	**1992**
Calcium	12 mg	10 mg
Iron	1.30 mg	103 mg
Magnesium	23 mg	23 mg
Phosphorus	203 mg	198 mg
Potassium	285 mg	238 mg
Vitamin A	150 I.U.	45 I.U.
Thiamine	0.100 mg	0.069 mg
Riboflavin	0.120 mg	0.134 mg
Niacin	7.70 mg	7.87 mg

Source: USDA, 1963[12] and 1997.[13]

Though there has been a general decline in minerals and vitamins over the years, some nutrient levels actually rose in some foods. The increase could be due to various factors: minerals in the fertilizers, supplements given to animals, or natural variations in the sampling methods. It is obvious that foods grown in different soils tend to have different mineral content. Phosphorus and potassium declined the least because they are added to fertilizers. The fact that iron declined the most is quite disturbing since other trace elements are not measured and may follow iron's decline.

ORGANIC VS. COMMERCIALLY GROWN FOODS

Due to the ever-growing presence of toxins in the environment, more people are opting for organically grown foods. Whether organically grown fruits, vegetables, and grains are more nutritious than chemically grown food has been a topic of scientific debate.[14] Many variables exist when comparing minerals of organic and commercially grown foods. First, studies usually compare only major minerals, excluding the three elements. Since major minerals are often added with chemical fertilizers, the amounts in commercial produce may be equal to or higher than those in organic crops. Second, averages from across the country do not give an accurate picture since mineral contents from different soils vary.

In 1993, a survey in Chicago was done comparing organic and conventional foods in supermarkets. It carefully paired up foods of the same variety and size at the same time of year.[15]

Table 4.4

Nutrients in Organic vs. Commercial Foods

MINERAL	ORGANIC HIGHER	COMMERCIAL HIGHER
Boron	70%	
Calcium	68%	
Chromium	78%	
Copper	48%	
Iodine	73%	
Iron		59%
Magnesium	136%	
Manganese	138%	
Phosphorus	91%	
Potassium	125%	
Rubidium		28%
Selenium	390%	
Silicon	86%	
Sodium	159%	
Sulfur	20%	
Vanadium	80%	
Zinc		60%

Source: B.L. Smith, 1993.

On the average, the organic foods have about twice the mineral content of chemically fertilized ones. In other parts of the country, this data may differ; however, the trend appears obvious.

A GUIDE TO MINERALS

Celtic Sea Salt

Due to modern agricultural methods, the mineral content of foods has declined. Therefore, we must consider supplementing our pets with natural mineral sources and not pills. Natural Celtic Sea Salt™ is a most basic condiment as well as a staple food. This sea salt is obtained from the evaporation of the ocean's water without synthetic chemicals. No synthetic supplement can equal the wealth of minerals that natural Celtic Sea Salt™ supplies, regardless of how rich the synthetic's content or how precisely it is formulated.[16]

Celtic Sea Salt™ is harvested in Brittany, near the Celtic Sea in the northwest of France. Cold, active, north sea currents; large tides; and other marine climatic conditions create a unique mix of minerals. It is this combination of minerals that gives Celtic Sea Salt™ its special qualities. Common salt lacks many of the minerals provided by Celtic Sea Salt™ because, during the refining process, these minerals are removed. Celtic Sea Salt™ is slightly gray in color, while regular salt is white.

Table 4.5 shows a clear distinction between natural Celtic Sea Salt™ and refined table salt. It is interesting to note that sea salt is only 84 percent sodium and chloride, while refined salt is 97.5 percent. This may be the reason for sea salt's mild "salty" but delicious flavor.

Mammalian bodies contain three internal oceans that closely resemble the ionic balance of ocean water. Each one of these complex solutions surrounds and circulates through animal and human bodies. Comparative analysis shows that these fluids—blood plasma, lymphatic fluid, and extracellular fluid—are similar to seawater in their chemical composition. Medical and biological facts indicate that mammals need salt in order to perform basic physiological functions. Ocean salt contains all of the minerals and trace elements that both humans and animals require. These minerals make salt a vital necessity. In the salty environment of amniotic fluid, the embryo grows 3 billion times in weight. From the moment of conception on, we are never without the need for salt.

Table 4.5		
Comparison of the Mineral Element in Natural Celtic Sea Salt™ vs. Refined Salt		
	CELTIC SEA SALT™	**REFINED SALT**
GROUP 1 Sodium & chloride	84%	97.5%
GROUP 2 Sulfur, magnesium, calcium & potassium	14%	0%
GROUP 3 Carbon, bromine, silicon, nitrogen, ammonium, fluorine, phosphorus, iodine, boron & lithium	1.9997%	0%
GROUP 4 Argon, rubidium, copper, molyldemon, manganese, vanadium, cobalt, silver, zinc, chromium, germanium, bismuth, gold, selenium & tin	0.0003%	0%
GROUP 5 All chemical additives which bleach, prevent water absorption, stabilize iodine additives & maintain free flow	0%	2.5%

Source: Modified from Biological Transmutations by C. Louis Kervran (1988).[17]

Proper electrolyte balance in the body is achieved by maintaining a relatively high potassium content inside the cell and a high sodium concentration in the fluid outside the cell (extracellular fluid). Though potassium and sodium are the two electrolytes found in the greatest concentration in the body, many other elements are required for normal physiological function. Trace elements bound in ocean water and in natural Celtic Sea Salt™ work to maintain proper function of the body's system. This unique combination of nutrients plays an important role in safeguarding good health. If any one element is left out or diminished, a link in an important chain will be missing and the whole organism will suffer. These elements work to regulate optimum body function by ensuring that the internal oceans are never shortchanged of trace nutrients.

At times, we find medical dogmas that have been around for many years and we are not exactly sure how they came about or what is the scientific basis for them. This dogma surrounds the controversy of low salt diets. Scientific research reveals that there are actually few salt-related health problems. A healthy, active lifestyle demands a sufficient and reasonable salt intake. The contention that our body can function on no salt at all or on a restricted ration of salt causes more problems than it is intended to solve. Life is closely dependent upon the presence of sodium. However, to clearly understand the role of sodium in blood, we must examine it in combination with water and various ions: chlorine, potassium, calcium, hydrogen, etc. It is more important to study the activity of sodium with these other ions, than to look at the sodium element alone. Most often in humans, salt-related health problems are caused by diets consisting of high quantities of refined sodium compounds, combined with a sedentary lifestyle.

Researchers at the Hypertension Center of the Cornell University Medical Center have shown that high blood pressure problems lie not in salt intake, but in an overactive hormone system.[18] When this system is overactive, renin levels are excessively high indicating a physiological need for salt. On the other hand, low-renin levels, which occur only in a third of hypertensive patients, actually reveal a sodium excess. Only these patients should be on a lower sodium intake. Factors that influence blood pressure are heart rate, changes in blood volume, and the constriction and dilation of blood vessels. A change in any one of these factors, providing the other two remain constant, will have a direct affect on blood pressure. Blood pressure regulation is achieved via the dilation and constriction of blood vessels (vasodilation/vasocon-striction) as well as the control of blood volume and heart rate. A healthy cardiovascular system may be maintained through regular exercise and proper weight.

Boron

Boron plays a role in bone metabolism. Though not totally clear, it seems to increase calcium absorption and utilization and reduces the amount of calcium and magnesium lost through the urine. Boron is necessary for action of vitamin D, the vitamin that stimulates the absorption and utilization of calcium. It may act by influencing the parathyroid hormone (PTH), which regulates the calcium-to-phosphorus ratio in the body. It may also help convert vitamin D into its active form, which increases the absorption of calcium from the intestines and reduces its loss through the kidneys.[19]

It appears that boron may also play a role in keeping joints healthy. In Germany, boron supplementation has been used for osteoarthritis since the 1970s. In an open trial in humans, boron supplementation of 6-9 mgs daily produced effective relief in 90 percent of arthritis patients, including patients with osteoarthritis, juvenile arthritis, and rheumatoid arthritis.[20]

Natural sources of boron: legumes, fruits, and nuts.

Calcium

Calcium is the most abundant mineral in the body. In fact, it comprises as much as 2 percent of the body's total body weight. As much as 99 percent of the body's calcium is found in bones and teeth; the other 1 percent is imperative for many other essential bodily functions.

Calcium combines with phosphorus to create calcium phosphate crystals, which form the bulk of the bone matrix. These crystals are incredibly light and strong, packed together within the bone in a pattern similar to the densely packed carbon crystals that form diamonds.[21] In fact, pound for pound, bone is four times stronger than reinforced concrete. Bone is a dynamic living tissue that is constantly changing. Bone requires a constant interchange of nutritional and hormonal factors to maintain its integrity.

The 1 percent of calcium not concentrated in bones and teeth is essential for such life processes as the passage of fluids between cell walls, blood clotting, much of the body's enzymatic activity, release of neurotransmitters, energy production, immune function, muscle contraction, and regulation of heart beat. The Krebs cycle, the body's primary mode of energy production, is dependent upon calcium. Metabolic rates may well be determined by a combination of calcium and magnesium.[22]

Vitamin D is vital to calcium absorption from the intestinal tract and maintains blood levels essential for the proper mineralization of bone. The body makes its own vitamin D with exposure to sunlight, so one must monitor closely when vitamin D is taken with calcium supplementation—or toxic levels of calcium can build up in the blood.

Natural sources of calcium: kelp, cheese, dulse, turnip greens, collard, kale, goat's milk, Brewer's yeast, spinach, almonds, sardines with bones, and raw milk.[23]

Copper

Copper is an essential trace element involved in several enzymatic reactions in the body. The role of copper in the blood is similar to that of iron. Copper assists in the transport of iron and the formation of hemoglobin. Obviously, a deficiency can lead to anemia.[24]

Copper is also involved in the structural integrity of connective tissue throughout the body.[25] Collagen is responsible for the integrity of bone, skin, cartilage, and tendons. Copper is also important in the structure of elastin, a connective tissue that gives elasticity to blood vessels, lungs, and skin, allowing them to move and stretch with changes in pressure or movement. Myelin sheath, which protects nerve cells, is also dependent upon copper. Copper is also an important cofactor in the formation of super oxide desmutase (SOD), a powerful antioxidant.

Bedlington terriers have a genetic predisposition when the liver accumulates dietary copper; this results in progressive hepatopathy and eventual liver failure. I suspect the liver is missing a key enzyme, which would help the liver excrete copper. A high intake of ascorbic acid, zinc, and iron may decrease the absorption of copper in this disease.

Natural sources of copper: beef, liver, Brazil nuts, millet, peas, barley, shellfish, chicken, beans, and mushrooms.

Germanium

Although germanium has no known requirement for humans or animals, a synthetic organic compound of germanium known as Ge-132 is reported to cure a number of chronic diseases, including cancer.

Japan has taken the forefront of Ge-132 research. Reports indicate that germanium has been helpful in treating a broad range of problems, including liver disease, hepatitis, cancer, leukemia, cataracts, and heart problems.[26] In this country, we tend not to trust complementary therapies that have not gone through the so-called "acid test," namely, a double-blind placebo trial. However, many, if not most, medical breakthroughs have come about with anecdotes and empirical observation. Our scientific community demands expensive, scientific, and, at times, even cruel research before widespread use of a substance can be used.

There have been a number of studies confirming the benefits of Ge-132. One study in 1984 confirmed that organic germanium restores the normal function of T cells, B-lymphocytes, antibody-dependent cell toxicity, natural killer cell activity, and a number of antibody forming cells. Studies indicate that this compound has unique physiological activity while being free of toxic side effects. Organic germanium has the ability to modulate the immune system.[27]

According to scientists at the University of Texas Medical Branch, Ge-132 is an immuno-potentiating agent with low toxicity in animals and stimulates macrophages (white blood cells that ingest foreign particles and infectious microorganisms) in mice.[28]

In 1979, scientists at the Sadaki Institute in Tokyo tested Ge-132 against several different strains of liver cancer in rats. They reported prolonged survival in animals with transplanted tumors. They concluded that such anti-tumor activities were entirely due to the activation of the animal's immune system. They further stated that Ge-132 has no cytotoxicity or ability to kill cancer cells.[29]

Germanium has also been touted as a great tissue oxygenator. Cells use oxygen to perform their various functions. Though not totally understood, germanium seems to have an oxygen-sparing effect and has even been shown to lower the requirement of oxygen.

The single most important substance for life, oxygen, is a powerful immune stimulant. Hypoxia is a serious condition that occurs when oxygen supplies to cells and tissues are depleted. Symptoms of aging may resemble symptoms of hypoxia. It may be possible to slow the aging process by administration of Ge-132. Other symptoms of hypoxia are fatigue, acidosis, weakness, and increased susceptibility to infection and possibly cancer. Cancer cells prefer an anaerobic environment and by increasing tissue oxygenation, cancer cells may be inhibited.

I have seen many animals benefit from Ge-132 in a variety of ailments. They seem to respond in a short period of time. The skin and mucous membranes take on a healthy pink color, and the guardians say that their pets seem more "perky." As we learn more about immunity, we should come closer to understanding precisely how organic germanium works. Our knowledge of organic germanium increases daily, and as it does, we will find more ways to fight degenerative diseases as well as cancers.

> **Natural sources of germanium:** ginseng, aloe vera, chlorella, garlic, shiitake mushroom, pearl barley, and water chestnuts.

Potassium

Potassium, sodium, and chloride are electrolytes that conduct electricity when dissolved in water. These closely linked nutrients are always found in pairs. They are either positive as in sodium, potassium, and calcium to mention just a few, or negative as in chloride and phosphate. In general, a potassium deficiency is characterized by muscle weakness, fatigue, mental confusion, general weakness, panting, heart problems, and nerve conduction disturbances. A disease in cats called Hypokalemic polymyopathy is characterized by ventroflexion of the neck, weakness, and a stilted and stiff leg gait when walking. This disease may be seen more in Burmese and Abyssinians. These cats respond quite quickly to potassium supplementation and must be maintained on it for life.

Potassium is an important electrolyte and functions in the maintenance of water balance, acid-base balance, muscle and nerve cell function, heart function, and kidney and adrenal function. Most of the body's potassium is housed in cells, while most of the body's sodium is located outside the cells in blood and other body fluids. The famous sodium-potassium pump helps keep potassium inside cells and sodium outside of cells. If sodium is not pumped out, water accumulates in the cell, causing it to swell and ultimately burst. The sodium-potassium pump also maintains the electrical charge within the cell. An electrical charge is produced during nerve transmission and muscle contraction while potassium exits and sodium enters. As you can see, a potassium deficiency affects muscles and nerves. Some older dogs with a potassium deficiency may show trembling of hind legs (though there may also be other reasons for this as well). In humans, it was shown that a high potassium, low sodium diet protects against cardiovascular disease, high blood pressure, cancer, and stroke.[30, 31]

Natural sources of potassium: bananas, avocado, lima beans, tomato, potato, cantaloupe, chicken, and fish.

Iodine

Iodine, a trace element, along with tyrosine, an amino acid, is required for the manufacture of thyroid hormones. A deficiency of iodine, though difficult to document, probably exists in some hypothyroid dogs. Symptoms of hypothyroidism in dogs are sluggishness, dull hair coat, weight gain, increased cholesterol, and generalized malaise. In people, a goiter is seen in the neck area where the thyroid enlarges to compensate for the decreased iodine intake. Some goiters are not due to a simple iodine deficiency. Over activity of the thyroid gland is called hyperthyroidism. In cats this is sometimes accompanied by a goiterous swelling. In humans, it is called Graves' Disease.[32] In both, the condition is life threatening with a sharp increase in metabolism. We will discuss treatments for thyroid disorders in chapter 10, which covers endocrine diseases.

Natural sources of iodine: kelp, Celtic Sea Salt™, dulse, sardines, herring, cod, and halibut.

Magnesium

Magnesium plays a major role in energy production and activates at least three hundred different enzymes. Magnesium is second only to potassium in terms of concentration within body cells. There is an intimate relationship between magnesium and calcium within the body. When magnesium is low, blood becomes saturated with calcium, which may deposit in the muscles or kidneys. Kidney stones may develop with prolonged low magnesium diets. Chronic vomiting, diarrhea, and prolonged use of diuretics can all predispose an animal to magnesium deficiency. Signs of magnesium deficiency are fatigue, irritability, muscle weakness, heart disturbances, muscle spasm, and nerve conduction problems.

I am concerned with commercial cat foods that contain low magnesium and which may lead to calcium oxalate crystals in the bladder. Research studies have reported that magnesium is a cause of bladder stones in cats; when in reality, it was the urine pH that was the determining factor and not magnesium.[33, 34] When cats were fed a diet containing magnesium chloride, an acidifying salt, no crystals were noted. However, when cats ingested a diet containing magnesium oxide, an alkalizing salt, struvite crystals were formed. This study confirmed that urinary acidification can minimize the rash of struvite formation and that magnesium was of less importance.

> **Natural sources of magnesium:** kelp, wheat bran, fish, meat, raw milk, green leafy vegetables, whole grains, and nuts.

Selenium

Selenium is an essential, nonmetallic trace element. It is called a "trace" mineral because it is needed in minute amounts. The body must have selenium, yet it cannot manufacture the element. Therefore, selenium must be supplied through the diet.

Food sources of selenium are directly related to soil levels of the element when the food is grown. These soil levels vary greatly from region to region throughout the world, ranging from a total lack of selenium to toxic levels as seen earlier in this century in the American West when livestock ate "locoweed," which were plants high in selenium. But experts agree that with each passing year, selenium levels have been declining and as such major diseases are increasing.[35]

The importance of selenium is that it functions primarily as a component of the antioxidant enzyme glutathione peroxidase, which works with vitamin E in preventing free radical damage to cell membranes. Low levels of selenium are linked to higher risks of cancer, cardiovascular disease, inflammatory disease, and other conditions associated with increased free-radical damage.[36, 37, 38]

Without adequate quantities of selenium, man and animals are more susceptible to cancer, virus, and free radical damage. Selenium is one of the most potent free radical scavengers that we call antioxidants. Selenium deficiency causes poor resistance to infectious organisms and reduces T cell activity and antibody production. Imagine an immune system that is unable to immobilize its T cells and natural killer cells to destroy pathogenic bacteria and viruses.[39] This is exactly what occurs in a selenium deficient immune system. A study in 1996, done on humans with HIV, found that the HIV virus replicated more rapidly in cells deficient in glutathione peroxidase.[40] Selenium supplementation was also found to increase interleuken-2, which is important in activating natural killer cell activity.[41] Interleuken-2 increased the rate of white blood cell proliferation and differentiation into forms capable of killing viruses and tumor cells.

A study involving humans with rheumatoid arthritis showed that selenium supplementation is important in reducing the production of inflammatory prostaglandins and leukotriene, as well as free radicals, factors that are thought to cause most of the damage seen in rheumatoid arthritis.[42]

Recent research also shows that selenium plays a role in the conversion of the thyroid hormone T4 into the metabolically active form, T3. Therefore, selenium deficiency may be partially implicated in some types of hypothyroidism.[43]

Natural sources of selenium: kelp, Brazil nuts, wheat germ, garlic, and seafood. I prefer to use kelp because it contains other trace elements such as zinc, magnesium, iodine, and other minerals that work in a synergistic manner.

Sulfur and Methyl-sulfonylmethane

So little is written on this compound that most people would be surprised that it is the third most plentiful mineral in both humans and animals. In fact, sulfur is found throughout the body and is included in the structure of proteins. It is an important component of many enzymes, hormones, and antibodies. As such, it is also organic, as opposed to inorganic. Two of the B vitamins, biotin and thiamine, contain sulfur.[44] Sulfur is especially abundant in the skin, hair, and nails, but its functions throughout the body are varied. It is part of the antioxidant enzyme glutamine peroxidase as well as the amino acids taurine, cystine, and methionine.[45]

MSM, short for methyl-sulfonylmethane, is a nutrient form of sulfur found in many common foods. MSM is not a medicine, drug, or food additive. It is a natural form of organic sulfur found in all living organisms. The body uses MSM to regenerate healthy tissues. Vitamins and amino acids work with MSM to achieve optimum health.

MSM is found in all foods; however, due to its unstable nature, MSM is quickly lost from food when it is processed, cooked, or stored. The second a fruit or vegetable is picked from a tree or vine, it rapidly loses its MSM.[46]

When an animal or human uses an MSM molecule to produce a new cell, that MSM is spent. The body must continually replenish its MSM bank to produce new, healthy cells. Processed foods do not supply enough MSM for optimum health. Because it is a free radical and foreign protein scavenger, MSM cleans the blood stream so allergies to food and pollens are eliminated in several days. Because of its short-lived nature, MSM should be taken daily.

Basically, one cannot overdose on MSM because the body will take and use whatever it needs. Approximately half of the total body sulfur is concentrated in the muscles, skin, and bones. It is present in keratin, the tough substance in the skin, nails, and hair. Sulfur is necessary for making collagen, the primary constituent of cartilage and connective tissue. It is responsible for the conformation of body proteins through the formation of disulfide bond, which holds connective tissue together.

Lacking sufficient MSM, the body is a compromised system, deficient in its ability to repair or replace damaged tissue or organs. The inability of the body to do its work causes it to produce dysfunctional cells, which can lead to disease.

Have you ever heard of anyone predicting weather changes because of pain they feel in their joints? Often, what contributes to the pain is the lack of flexibility and permeability in the fibrous tissue cells. Use of MSM has been shown to add flexibility to cell walls while allowing fluids to pass through the tissue more easily. MSM softens the tissues and helps to equalize pressure, thereby reducing pain. This important property of MSM can help treat a wide variety of conditions. Many types of pain can be attributed to pressure differential involving cells that make up tissue. When outside pressure drops, cells inflate and become inflamed. Nerves register the inflammation, and pain is experienced.[47]

MSM can serve as a dietary source of sulfur. Remember that MSM is a natural form of organic sulfur found in all living organisms and present in low concentrations in body tissues. Only fresh and raw unprocessed foods contain MSM. MSM has been found to normalize certain body functions in patients displaying physiological symptoms of stress, specifically gastrointestinal upset, inflammation of mucous membranes, allergic reactions, constipation, muscle cramps, infectious parasites, and arthritis.[48]

Flexibility between cells is in part attributed to MSM. It acts to block undesirable chemical and physiological cross-linking or bonding of collagen, which is associated with tough, aging skin. Therefore, MSM enhances tissue pliability and encourages the repair of damaged skin. If insufficient MSM is ingested, then newly produced skin cells become rigid. The rigidity can contribute to cracking, wrinkles, and scar tissue. When sufficient MSM is present, it surfaces to make the skin softer, smoother, and more flexible, allowing it to stretch easily with movement. Vitamin C, which is also required for the production of collagen, is abundant in a variety of fruits and vegetables. Clearly, MSM offers a broad range of health benefits to humans and pets, and should be part of a comprehensive fresh raw diet.

> **Natural sources of MSM:** fruits, vegetables, meat, fish, milk, and eggs. Animal protein foods contain higher amounts of this compound, particularly eggs.

Zinc

Zinc is found in virtually every cell in the body and is a component in more than two hundred enzymes. It is also important for the proper action of many hormones, such as thyroid, insulin, sex, growth, and thymic hormones.[49]

Zinc is involved in many aspects of the immune system, but particularly the thymus gland. The thymus gland is to the immune system what a general is to an army. Without a healthy thymus gland, the immune system can't do the job its suppose to do. Zinc is the most important mineral to the thymus gland. When zinc levels are low, the number of T cells decreases, thymic hormone levels drop, and many white blood cell functions critical for the immune response stop. Fortunately, zinc supplementation can rejuvenate the thymus gland.[50]

Zinc is essential for proper cell growth and replication. It is required for protein synthesis and, therefore, rapid wound healing. It is also essential for reproduction, vision, taste, and smell. A zinc deficiency results in impaired function of these senses.

The importance of zinc in normal skin function is well known. Zinc responsive dermatosis in dogs is well publicized.[51] These dogs may have difficulty in absorbing zinc, perhaps through a genetic malfunction. They no doubt have a defect in cell mediated immunity due to a depressed thymus gland. But as stated earlier, the thymus gland can rejuvenate with proper zinc supplementation.

Natural sources of zinc: oysters, shellfish, kelp, fish, red meat, whole grains, legumes, nuts, and seeds. However, zinc in plant foods is less available because it binds to phytic acid.

chapter 5

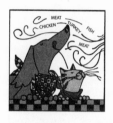

Raw Meat Diets and the Enzyme Connection

BEFORE DISCUSSING VARIOUS DIETS, IT IS IMPORTANT to discuss raw meat and the importance of enzymes. There is convincing evidence derived from the works of Drs. Francis Pottinger,[1] Weston Price,[2] and Edward Howell[3] that the destruction of enzymes found in food plays a significant role in chronic degenerative diseases in both humans and animals. It begins with a destructive process known as digestive leukocytosis. "Leukocytosis" is a pathological condition that *Dowlands Illustrated Medical Dictionary* defines as "a transient increase in the number of leukocytes in the blood, resulting from various causes such as hemorrhage, fever, infection, inflammation, etc."

Leukocytosis was first discovered in 1846. At first, it was considered normal because everyone who was tested had it. Dr. Paul Kantchakoff, however, later found that leukocytosis was a pathological condition.[4] In fact, the major cause of leukocytosis was discovered to be the eating of cooked food. An entire category of leukocytosis was classified as "digestive leukocytosis," that is, the elevation of the white blood cell level in response to the lack of enzymes in the cooked food in the intestine. It is pathological because the pancreas was never intended to provide 100 percent of the digestive enzymes needed. I believe digestive leukocytosis is more prevalent than food allergies.

Kantchakoff divided his findings into four classifications according to the severity of the pathological reaction in the blood:

1. Raw food produced no increase in the white blood cell count.

2. Commonly cooked food caused leukocytosis.

3. Pressure-cooked food caused even greater leukocytosis.

4. Man-made, processed, and refined foods, such as carbonated beverages, alcohol, vinegar, white sugar, flour, and other foods, caused severe leukocytosis. Cooked, smoked, and salted animal meat brought on violent leukocytosis consistent with ingesting poison.

This phenomenon occurs after eating cooked food, since prolonged heat above 118 degrees F destroys enzymes in food. Three minutes in boiling water destroys 80 to 95 percent of the enzymes in food, while baking, frying, broiling, stewing, and canning destroys 100 percent of enzymes. Nature designed food to have sufficient enzymes to digest the food when it is ingested. When enzymes are destroyed by cooking or other processing, ingested enzyme-deficient food triggers the body's immune system, which responds with leukocytosis. Remember how you felt after eating a large Thanksgiving meal; that's "digestive leukocytosis." Your body is dumping enzymes from its "enzyme bank" to digest its food. This process puts significant stress on the pancreas, accounting for enlarged pancreas and the proliferation of chronic degenerative diseases. Some researchers suggest that the dwindling supply of enzymes in humans and animals not only leads to illness, but also to death.[5]

The medical dictionary defines an enzyme as a protein produced in a cell capable of accelerating, by its catalytic action, the chemical reaction of a substance for which it is specific. In a nutshell, enzymes are the body's workers. Enzymes operate on a biological and chemical level, and although vitamins, minerals, hormones, proteins, and other substances are essential to life, it is the enzymes that perform the work and utilize these substances in restoring, repairing, and maintaining health and life. Without enzymes, life would not exist. In fact, when enzyme levels fall below a given level in any living system, life ceases.[6] Man has attempted and failed to produce synthetic enzymes. It took nature millions of years to produce enzymes, and she is not about to reveal this secret. Man and animals replenish their enzyme systems with the ingestion of raw unprocessed food.

As stated before, enzymes are delicate compounds responsible for nearly every chemical reaction that occurs in the body. Digestion and all metabolic pathways rely on enzymes to function. Enzymes are found in all living cells, both plants and animals, and are therefore found in food. Enzymes participate in at least 80,000 enzyme systems in the body. In fact, many researchers suggest that the enzyme is the substance we call "life force." The significance of enzymes in the diet has by and large been ignored by physicians, nutritionists, and veterinarians. It is commonly believed that enzymes, being protein molecules, are broken down by digestion and are therefore of no more importance than any other protein in the food. However, various significant pieces of evidence point to the understanding that enzymes within food itself can survive intact in the digestive tract, thus sparing excess bodily exertion needed to secrete enzymes for digestive processes.[7] In fact, the continued eating of enzyme-less processed food places a chronic extra demand upon the limited enzyme potential of the body, which leads to disease and eventual death.[8]

Enzymes do things that in a laboratory requires up to 2,000 degrees F to duplicate. They are present in raw food in direct proportion to the proteins, complex carbohydrates, lipids, and other food constituents that exist there. Food enzymes break food down so its constituents are small enough to pass into the blood or lymph system, enabling the body to effectively utilize them. It is important to emphasize that eating raw unprocessed foods contain the enzymes in exact proportions needed for the digestion of that particular food.[9] Thus, enzymes prevent the body from tapping its "enzyme bank" to keep the body healthy and free of disease. Fifty years of research on enzyme nutrition by Dr. Edward Howell suggests that animals and humans are born with a finite amount of enzymes, and when the "enzyme bank" is depleted, death ensues. Modern high-heat processed foods contribute nothing to the digestive system and force the body to provide all digestive enzymes. It is therefore reasonable to expect that not only will food be incompletely digested, but that the continual one-sided effort of the body to secrete enzymes would eventually take its toll on digestive organs. This constant pressure on the pancreas causes it to enlarge, weaken, and eventually atrophy. It has been shown by Howell that the pancreas of wild mice weighed one-third of that found in mice raised in laboratories on processed lab chow.[10]

It was once believed that because enzymes can be produced by the body, there could never be a deficiency. However, not only enzymes but other essential biochemicals normally synthesized by the body, such as certain amino acids, vitamins, and necessary nutrients, can become deficient. It has now been established that the number of enzymes the body can produce in a lifetime is limited. Therefore, it is important to add enzymes through raw foods and enzyme supplementation to human and animal diets. This will allow the limited number of endogenous enzymes to last much longer since, according to the "law of adoptive secretion," the pancreas will only secrete the amount necessary.

Due to modern food processing, packaging, and preparation that make longer shelf life possible, prepared food is essentially "dead" relative to animal nutritional needs. An animal can exist on packaged foods; however, such a diet may take its toll on good health. Enzyme-rich raw food diets and their positive effects on various diseased conditions in both humans and animals have been well documented throughout the world. The first major scientific paper on enzymes was published on April 15, 1940, by Howell in the *Journal of the American Association for Medico-Physical Research*. He pioneered more than fifty years of research and scientific experimentation with overwhelming evidence indicating that the primary cause of degenerative disease in humans and animals is enzyme deficiency exacerbated by enzyme deficient mothers passing on genetic deficiencies to their offspring.

In the early 1930s and over the following twenty-five years, Dr. Francis Pottinger conducted studies on cats using two diets. One diet consisted of two-thirds raw meat and one-third raw milk and cod liver oil. The second diet consisted of two-thirds cooked meat and one-third raw milk and cod liver oil. The results of the studies were significant. Multiple generations of cats on the raw meat diet were healthy. They had adequate nasal cavities, excellent tissue tone, good fur with little shedding, and no facial deformities. The calcium and phosphorus content of their bones was consistent. Throughout their life spans, they were resistant to infections, fleas, and other parasites. They were free of allergies, and miscarriages were rare. They were quite healthy.

On the other hand, the multiple generations of cats on the cooked meat diets were not so healthy. They had many variations in facial bone and dental structure. Their long bones tended to be increased in length and smaller in diameter, showing less calcium. In the third generation, some of the bones were as soft as rubber. Other indications were heart problems, visual problems, thyroid problems, gland problems, kidney problems, arthritis, various infections, and neurologic diseases. Infections of the bone appeared regularly, often appearing to be the cause of death. By the time the third generation was born, the cats were so physically compromised that none survived beyond six months of age. Cats on the cooked meat diet were also more unstable. Pneumonia was a principal cause of death in adult cats, while diarrhea was the cause in the deaths of kittens. Many reproductive problems were also observed.

It is interesting to note that when cats from the first and second generation groups that had been fed cooked meat were returned to a raw meat diet, it took about four generations to recover a state of normal health. Improvement in resistance to disease was noted in the second generation, with allergic manifestations persisting in the third generation. By the fourth generation, most of the severe deficiency symptoms disappeared, but seldom completely. Once these kittens were put on an optimum diet, their disease processes reversed.

Howell made interesting observations when studying more than 3,000 Arctic Eskimos. Their main diet consisted of raw meat and fat. They and their sled dogs ate the same diet, and both were disease free. Only one Eskimo in 3,000 was slightly overweight. You are probably thinking that their physical lifestyle may have contributed to their health. Well, that may only be a small part of the reason. It turns out that Cathepsin and lipase, a muscle and fat enzyme, respectively, within the raw food, assist the body in digestion, thus sparing the body from having to use up endogenous enzymes. It is important to understand that enzymes within raw food digest the food itself. This is the reason Eskimos are not overweight.

In the wild, animals on their natural diets are relatively free of degenerative disease. When animals are put on processed diets, two things consistently occur: the animal's life span is cut by as much as 185 percent and its weight increases by as much as 164 percent. Animals on processed diets have lower brain weight than their wild counterparts who must search for food. This has been seen in mice in captivity on standard lab chow diets.

Every dog or cat, regardless of the diet, should be supplemented with enzymes to replenish the body's "enzyme bank." Because the nutrient levels of foods are depleted by pesticides, growing conditions, poor soil, processing, storage, and cooking, enzyme supplementation is imperative. But remember, enzyme supplements are only an adjunct to a natural raw food diet and not a substitute.

A GUIDE TO ENZYME SUPPLEMENTS

- **Papain:** Obtained from the papaya plant. It helps in malabsorption syndrome.

- **Bromelain:** From the stem of the pineapple plant. It is a sulfur containing compound and reduces inflammation.

- **Protease:** From animal, plant, and microbial sources. This enzyme hydrolyzes proteins to amino acids.

- **Amylase:** From animal, plant, and microbial sources. It breaks down starch into digestible carbohydrates.

- **Lipase:** Also from a variety of sources and dependent on calcium ions. Lipase splits emulsified neutral fats into fatty acids and glycerol.

- **Lactase:** From yeast or fungal sources. It helps with lactose intolerance.

- **Cellulase:** From Aspergillus mold. It breaks down cellulose, the fibrous membrane of plant foods. The gastrointestinal tract lacks any enzyme capable of hydrolyzing cellulose, and so, cellulose goes undigested. The importance of the ability to digest cellulose is in allowing essential nutrients found within this structural compound to be released and utilized.

ENZYMES IN FOOD

By supplementing with exogenous enzymes to the diet, a number of benefits occur. First, enhanced enzymatic digestion in the stomach results in increased digestion and absorption of nutrients with less undigested product passing with the stool.[11] Other benefits include larger litters, better weight management, improved skin condition, resistance to stress, and decreased food sensitivities and allergies.[12, 13]

Table 5.1	
Enzymes in Foods	
FOOD	**ENZYMES**
Apple	Peroxidase
Banana	Amylase, maltase, sucrase
Corn	Amylase
Egg	Tributyrinase, lipase, phosphatase, peptidase, peroxidase, catalase, oxidase, amylase
Kidney Beans	Amylase, Protease
Meat	Cathepsin
Raw Milk	Catalase, Galactase, Lactase, Amylase, Oleinase, Peroxidase, Dehydrogenase, Phosphatase, lipase
Potato	Invertase
Raw honey	Amylase, catalase
Sugar Cane	Amylase, Catalase, Ereptase, Invertase, Maltase, Oxidase, Peroxidase, Peptase, Saccharase, Tryosinase
Wheat	Amylase, Protease
Rice	Amylase

Source: Howell, E., *Enzyme Nutrition* (1985).

The enzymes in these foods correspond to the nutrients that must be digested in the foods and, thus, alleviate the need for the body's enzymes to do the digestion. As can be seen, raw milk is loaded with healthful enzymes, and if you are able to obtain it, then by all means, drink it in good health and don't forget your furry little loved ones. Raw cow's milk is almost a perfect food, and in the future, it will be more widely available. I drink raw milk daily and feel great when I drink it. My pets get it daily as well. There is a lot of misinformation about raw milk, and the only problem is that it is not more widely available. I have never become ill from the ingestion of raw milk, but I am allergic to pasteurized milk. Certified raw milk is more resistant to putrifaction then pasteurized milk and contains vitamins A, B-complex, C, D, and E; a host of minerals; and at least thirty enzymes. This is truly medicine from nature, and we destroy it by pasteurization.

ENZYME INHIBITORS

With all the talk about enzymes and raw foods, I must discuss the subject of enzyme inhibitors. Grains such as wheat, soy, barley, corn, and rice are used extensively, but knowledge of their food enzymes is less widespread. In the grain family, more is known about barley enzymes because barley is used in the brewing industry. Barley is germinated or sprouted by the malting process, in which the enzymes, particularly amylase, increase.

Any seed can be made to germinate by boiling in water. Resting seeds contain starch, which is a storage nutrient and a source of future energy when conditions become ideal for the seed to germinate and grow into a plant. In nature, seeds must rest for months or years before conditions become satisfactory for them to grow. Enzymes are present in the resting seed but are prevented from being active by the presence of enzyme inhibitors. Germination neutralizes the inhibitors and releases the enzymes. These enzyme inhibitors must be neutralized before ingested, or they will stop endogenous enzymes from functioning. It is obvious that enzyme inhibitors are needed only in the seeds and not in other parts of the plant. But what is required for the well-being of seeds poses problems for animals and humans wanting to eat the seeds for food. In the forest, squirrels make a practice of burying nuts in the ground and digging them up for food after they have germinated. Not all the nuts will be eaten, and the ones that are not may grow into trees. This is the way animals naturally adapt to circumvent enzyme inhibitors in the wild.

CATS AND TAURINE

It is also important to note that cooking meat destroys taurine. Natural taurine in raw meat is essential for the well-being and health of cats. Adding isolated taurine to processed foods may prevent acute problems—but not chronic problems—in many cats. I believe that cats have a high affinity for natural taurine from foods. Lack of natural taurine may contribute to the chronic kidney failure we see in cats. Taurine has antioxidant effects and, in cats, I believe has special affinity not only to the heart and eyes, but also the kidneys.

Table 5.2		
Taurine Content of Selected Foods		
FOOD	**RAW**	**BOILED**
Beef muscle	362	60
Beef liver	192	73
Beef kidney	225	76
Lamb muscle	473	126
Lamb kidney	239	51
Pork muscle	496	118
Pork liver	169	43
Chicken muscle	337	82
Cod	314	161
Oysters	698	89
Clams	2400	446

Source: Wysong, R.L., *Rationale for Animal Nutrition* (Inquiry Press, 1998).[14]

This is only a partial list of food items with taurine content, and one can alternate food items from time to time to make meals more interesting and palatable. Remember that diets provided in this chapter are only a guideline and not a hard and fast rule. Your individual pet's needs, lifestyle, and palatability requirements should all be taken into consideration. Today's busy owners seem always on the run and find it difficult to cook for themselves much less their pets. However, I believe that we can all add some natural raw foods to our pets' processed "dead" foods. If you don't want to give raw meat daily, then trying giving it to your pet every other day.

RAW EGGS: THE PERFECT FOOD

Raw eggs are practically a perfect food, just as raw milk is. You can give your pet raw eggs, preferably from cage-free chickens. By giving the whole egg, including the white, you don't have to worry about biotin deficiency. It is a myth that raw egg whites will cause biotin deficiency.

DOGS AND CATS HAVE LITTLE NUTRITIONAL NEED FOR GRAINS

Dogs and cats have no nutritional needs for grains, and food manufacturers use them as a filler. Some grains, though highly nutritious, should be fed at no more than 10 percent of the total diet. Various cooked whole grains such as amaranth, barley, brown rice, oats, quinta, buckwheat, and millet can be used. Wheat germ, which is a great source of natural vitamin E complex, can also be given. Diabetic animals should never be fed grains, as this will exacerbate hyperglycemia.

DIETS

Raw Meat

Pets can be given raw beef, chicken, lamb, and turkey as well as organ meats such as liver, heart, or kidney. Remember, cats need preformed vitamin A that is obtained from liver. Liver can be given to cats two to three times per week in small amounts. Raw eggs can be substituted for meat as a change of pace. Occasionally, fresh fish and sardines may be given to cats for variety. Add ¼ cup for each 10 pounds body weight.

Raw Vegetables

Vegetables may be given raw: chopped, grated, or lightly steamed. Experiment to see which vegetables your pet finds palatable. Try carrots, zucchini, garlic, broccoli, romaine lettuce, green beans, kale, okra, parsley, squash, broccoli, sprouts, red pepper, and celery. Many pets also enjoy some fruit at times. Dogs can be fed ⅛ to ¼ cup of vegetables for each 10 pounds. Feed cats 1 to 2 tablespoons per 10 pounds.

Raw Bone

Carnivores in the wild eat raw bone, and this is much better absorbed than cooked bone meal. Cooked bone can splinter and cause serious intestinal problems. No such problems are seen with raw bones. They also help keep teeth clean. Raw chicken and turkey necks are a good source of calcium. Chicken backs are also acceptable. Large dogs enjoy beef knuckle bones. Cats must have their bones cut a bit more finely than do dogs.

Add ½ to 1 chicken neck per 10-pound body weight.

Celtic Sea Salt™

Feed pets ¼ to ½ teaspoon per meal.

Kelp

Feed pets ⅛ teaspoon to 1 teaspoon per meal.

Flax Seed Oil

Dogs can be fed ½ to 1 tablespoon once or twice daily. Cats do not find flax oil as palatable as dogs. However, they will accept crushed flax seed and can be given ¼ to ½ teaspoon per meal.

Food Concentrates

There are also various food concentrates in the marketplace that contain natural vitamins and that can be used to supplement the diet. I have formulated a natural food concentrate, which contains freeze-dried raw bone meal, alfalfa, carrot powder, brown rice bran, nutritional yeast, oat flour, peavine juice, garlic, broccoli, sprouts, ascerola berry, potato flour, adrenal, liver, spleen, kidney, kelp, beet root, and carob. I do not recommend synthetic vitamins in any form as a supplement. They will only add an unneeded burden on your pet to detoxify. Only natural nutrients from foods should be given.

KEEP IT SIMPLE

Remember, natural nutrients from food sources go a long way toward optimum health. Experimenting to see what is palatable is a natural occurrence when providing raw diets. Pets must get acclimated slowly to any diet. Many pets find beef and chicken broth palatable; both can be added to the diet. Remember, no processed "dead" food is 100 percent complete, regardless of whether the food has a natural sounding name. You can make that processed food more complete by adding your "live" homemade raw food diet.

When feeding pets, humans seem to insist on making elaborate menus as if they were a chef in a restaurant. I am reminded of an old acronym: KISS or keep it simple, stupid. Nature in her evolutionary genius designed nutrients as "package deals." It only became complicated and unwholesome when modern man decided to change nature's gift of nutrients.

WHAT DO PETS REALLY NEED?

Carbohydrates

Pets do not need dietary carbohydrates from grain sources. They provide the most calories in commercial pet foods and are the least expensive. The only grains wild cats or dogs ingest is from the stomachs of their prey. High carbrohydrate-based diets may over-tax the pancreas and may make pets prone to diabetes, pancreatitis, and other degenerative diseases.

Fats

Fats are necessary for good health and disease prevention. Here again, fats should be raw or unrefined—not processed. Meat, fish, eggs, or milk in their natural states are the best sources of fat. The pet food industry prepares some pet foods with high levels of omega-3 fatty acids that are claimed to be effective for treating various inflammatory diseases. However, omega-3 fatty acids are quite sensitive to heat and are destroyed and easily become rancid during processing. Cod liver oil can be added to pet foods. It is a good source of omega-3 fatty acids as well as vitamin A.

Proteins

Proteins are the most costly and important ingredient in your pet's food diet. Remember, cereal grains do not provide all of the required amino acids. Raw meat in the form of chicken, beef, lamb, fish, and turkey are good sources of protein. Raw eggs from cage-free chickens, especially chickens fed blue-green algae or flax to increase their omega-3 fatty acids, are also excellent protein sources. It is also important to provide a variety of organ meats as well.

Cats require preformed vitamin A, which is found in liver. Raw liver can be safely fed two or three times a week. Pets are more resistant to salmonella or E.coli problems than are humans. The benefits of feeding pets raw meat far outweigh any potential digestive disturbances. If possible, purchase meat at a reliable health food store or supermarket.

The problem of parasites in raw meat in the United States is minimal but easily solved by freezing meat for fourteen days. Raw fish, however, loses its firmness and texture when frozen. To kill parasites in raw fish, marinate or ferment the fish in an acid solution of lemon juice, lime juice, or whey. This will predigest the fish as well. It is interesting that modern man living in industrialized societies is concerned about eating raw meat and fish, while Eskimos who lived off of raw meat, blubber, and fish were not plagued by food poisoning or degenerative diseases. The Eskimos learned to live with nature and were rewarded with health and vitality.

CAT DIETS

Beef Diet (range fed)

¼–½ cup raw ground beef

¼–½ teaspoon Celtic Sea Salt™ or kelp

1 teaspoon raw beef liver

1 teaspoon cod liver oil

¼ raw chicken neck, finely chopped, or one calcifood wafer from standard process

Chicken Diet (cage free)

¼–½ cup raw chicken or giblets

¼–½ teaspoon Celtic Sea Salt™ or kelp

1 teaspoon raw chicken liver

1 tablespoon vegetables, finely grated (parsley, carrots, zucchini, sprouts, kale, okra, green beans)

¼ raw chicken neck, chopped, or one calcifood wafer

Turkey Diet (organically raised)

¼–½ cup raw ground turkey

¼–½ teaspoon Celtic Sea Salt™ or kelp

1 teaspoon raw beef liver

1 teaspoon cod liver oil

¼ raw chicken neck, chopped, or one calcifood wafer

Lamb Diet (range fed)

¼–½ cup raw ground lamb
¼–½ teaspoon Celtic Sea Salt™ or kelp
1 teaspoon raw beef liver
1 tablespoon finely grated vegetables
¼ raw chopped chicken neck, or one calcifood wafer
1 teaspoon cod liver oil

Fish Diet

1 can sardines with bones in olive oil
1 tablespoon finely grated vegetables
1 tablespoon clam juice

Or
½ can sardines with bones in olive oil
2 tablespoons raw marinated fish (salmon, trout, herring, mackerel, tuna)
1 teaspoon cod liver oil

Or
2 tablespoons raw shrimp, crab, lobster
1 tablespoon finely grated vegetables
¼ raw chopped chicken neck, or one calcifood wafer
1 teaspoon cod liver oil

Egg Diet (cage free)

1 raw egg, beaten
¼–½ teaspoon Celtic Sea Salt™ or kelp
1 teaspoon finely grated vegetables
¼ raw chopped chicken neck, or one calcifood wafer
1 teaspoon raw chicken or beef liver
1 teaspoon cod liver oil

These recipes are guidelines and must be customized for your individual pet's taste. Cats can be quite finicky, so experimenting with the palatability of various menus is a must. One may add raw meat to palatable canned food or broth that does not contain onion powder. Use your imagination and experiment to be successful.

A final comment on concerns about raw milk: If one has access to it, I strongly urge you to give raw milk to your pet. It is a complete protein sources as well as a source of calcium. If you give your cat raw milk, then chicken necks and calcifood wafer is unnecessary.

DOG DIETS

Dogs are much easier to feed than cats. Palatability is much less of an issue with dogs than it is with cats. Though dogs are carnivores, they can be fed more vegetable matter per body weight than cats. The following recipes are guidelines. Feel free to experiment with various vegetables, meats, fish, eggs, and organ meats. Keep in mind that organ meats possess more vitamins than muscle meats.

It is important to vary your dog's diet from time to time as various foods contain different nutrients. Like humans, pets grow tired of the same foods day in and day out.

Last but not least, remember that raw bones are an important source of calcium as well as other nutrients for arthritic dogs. You may wonder why not feed bone meal? Bone meal is a cooked and processed product; processing has depleted its calcium content and destroyed its enzymes. It may also contain lead, which can cause disease.

Many large breed dogs do quite well consuming large beef knuckle bones, which help clean the teeth. The raw marrow is quite nutritious as well. Raw poultry bones from chickens, ducks, or turkeys are safe and will not splinter. Many dogs have done well on raw chicken necks and backs. At times, dogs may swallow a piece of bone that is too large and vomit it up. Don't be alarmed; they may need smaller pieces or just to become accustomed to it.

Beef Diet for Dogs

¼ cup/10 lbs. of raw beef (organ meats added)
1 raw chicken neck/10 lbs.
¼ teaspoon/10 lbs. Celtic Sea Salt™ or kelp
1 tablespoon/10 lbs. chopped vegetables
½ teaspoon/10 lbs. flax oil or crushed flax seeds
¼ teaspoon/10 lbs. cod liver oil

Chicken, lamb, turkey, duck, or fish may be substituted for beef in the above diet. Potatoes, if given, must be cooked with the skin left on. One may vary this diet occasionally by adding small amounts of cottage or cream cheese, cooked whole grains, or raw eggs (cage free). Remember, dogs have no requirement for whole grains, but many pet owners provide it because it is economical. By providing a varied diet, pets will consume a variety of nutrients needed for optimum health.

chapter 6

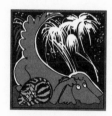

Enhancing the Immune System

THE IMMUNE SYSTEM IS A NETWORK OF CELLS AND ORGANS that defends the body against attacks by foreign invaders. The cells communicate with each other through proteins called cytokines to mount a defensive attack. The body is mainly being defended against what are popularly called germs or microbes (bacteria, yeast, protozoan, and viruses). Because the mammalian body provides an ideal environment (warmth and moisture) for many microbes, they tend to multiply easily and rapidly in the body if the immune system has been unable to keep them out or destroy them. Symptoms or illness may arise directly from the actions of the pathological organisms, from the immune system activities called upon to fight them, and/or both.

The immune system is amazingly complex. Every time we solve a problem, two more questions arise. The immune system must recognize dozens of different enemies and then produce secretions and "killer" cells to match up with and wipe out each one of them. But it gets even trickier: the immune system must produce this response only when the enemy is present; otherwise, the immune system would be draining energy and building up secretions continuously.

The secret to the immune system's success is an elaborate and dynamic communications network and memory. Millions and millions of cells of different types pass information back and forth like a swarm of bees. Once immune cells receive an alarm signal, they undergo strategic changes and begin to produce powerful chemicals. These substances allow the cells to regulate their own growth and behavior, enlist millions of similar cells, and direct newly recruited cells to the trouble spots. Unfortunately, with its complexity, the immune system can sometimes produce undesired effects, such as allergy and autoimmune responses. To begin to understand the immune system, it is necessary to learn the functions of several of its components.

STRUCTURE OF THE IMMUNE SYSTEM

The primary organs of the immune system are positioned throughout the body. They are called lymphoid organs because they are home to lymphocytes, small white blood cells that are key players in the immune system. Bone marrow, the soft tissue in the hollow center of bones, is the ultimate source of all blood cells, including the white blood cells destined to become immune cells.[1] If the lymphocyte-producing cells are inhibited by certain drugs, such as many of the anticancer drugs, then the amount of lymphocytes becomes relatively small, this is called leukopenia. On the other hand, if the lymphocyte-producing cells of the bone marrow become cancerous, huge amounts of white blood cells are produced. This condition is called leukemia.

The newly produced white blood cells are destined to mature into various types of functional immune cells. Some of the lymphocytes become B cells (B for bone marrow). Others migrate and mature in the thymus gland, a small organ that lies behind the breastbone; these are called T cells (T for thymus). A small proportion (less than 10 percent) of the white blood cells become natural killer cells (NK cells).

Lymphocytes can travel throughout the body, either through the blood vessels or the lymphatic vessels that carry lymph, a somewhat milky fluid that replenishes the blood with chyle (emulsified fat), erythrocytes (red blood cells), and leukocytes (white blood cells). Imagine small creeks that empty into larger and larger river channels. At the base of the neck, lymphocytes merge into two ducts—the thoracic duct and the right lymphatic duct—which discharge their contents into the bloodstream.

Small, bean-shaped lymph nodes are laced along the lymphatic vessels throughout the body. Each lymph node contains specialized compartments where immune cells congregate, and where they encounter antigens. An antigen is any substance that will elicit an immune response, so that the body will produce antibodies specific for that substance. During infections and some cancers, the lymph nodes may enlarge as they fill with immune cells and their targets.

The spleen is another part of the lymph system. It is a fist-sized organ at the upper right quadrant of the abdomen. Like the lymph nodes, the spleen contains specialized compartments where immune cells gather, and serves as a meeting ground where antigens and immune defenses interact.[2]

Clumps of lymphoid tissue are found in many parts of the body, especially in the linings of the digestive tract and the airways and lungs. Immune cells and foreign particles enter the lymph nodes via incoming lymphatic vessels or the tiny blood vessels that supply the lymph nodes. Lymphocytes exit the lymph nodes through outgoing lymph vessels. Once in the bloodstream, the lymphocytes are transported to tissues throughout the body. They gradually drift back into the lymphatic system to be cycled through again.

Phagocytes and Granulocytes

Phagocytes are large white blood cells that can engulf and digest microbes or other foreign particles. Monocytes are those phagocytes that are circulating in the blood. When monocytes migrate into tissues, they develop into macrophages. Specialized types of macrophages can be found in many organs, including the lungs, kidneys, liver, and brain.[3]

Macrophages play many roles. As scavengers, they rid the body of worn out cells and other debris. They display bits of foreign antigen in a way that makes it easy for the matching lymphocytes to become involved in the attack. They also churn out a group of cytokines, known as monokynes, that are vital to the immune responses. Cytokines allow cells to communicate with each other.

Granulocytes are yet another group of white blood cells that contain granules filled with biochemicals, which can destroy microorganisms. Some of these chemicals, such as histamine, also contribute to the inflammation process and allergy. One type of granulocyte, the neutrophil, is also a phagocyte; it uses its chemicals to degrade the microbes it ingests. Eosinophils and basophils are granulocytes that spray their chemicals onto harmful cells or microbes nearby. Most cells are similar to basophils, but are not blood cells. They are found in the lungs, skin, tongue, and linings of the nose and intestinal tract, where they are responsible for the symptoms of allergy as well as normal immune responses. A related structure is the cell fragment known as a blood platelet, which also contains granules. In addition to promoting blood clotting and wound repair, platelets activate some of the immune defenses.

Complement System
The complement system is made up of about twenty-five biochemicals that work together to complement the action of antibodies in destroying foreign cells and removing the antigen-antibody complexes (produced by B cells). An antigen-antibody complex is a specific combination composed of an antibody and an antigen (foreign substance, bacteria, virus, parasite). Proteins in the complement system can cause blood vessels to become dilated, and then leaky; this allows immune components to exit the blood and enter surrounding tissues. These components

contribute to the redness, warmth, swelling, pain, and loss of function that characterize the inflammatory response. Complement proteins circulate in the blood in an inactive form until the first protein in the system is activated by an antibody-antigen complex. Each component then takes its turn in a precise chain of steps known as the complement cascade.[4] The end product is a protein cylinder that punctures the wall of the cell under attack and serves as an open channel between the interior and exterior of the cell. The cell then swells up and bursts with its larger constituents taken up by macrophages.

Natural Killer Cells

Natural killer cells (NK cells) are the body's first line of defense against invading microbes. These cells also seek out and destroy on contact cancer cells before they find a place to attack and develop into a tumor. Like phagocytes, natural killer cells do not need to be told to deal with an invader or infected cell. They act independently on their own. Unlike other cells of the immune system, NK cells do not have memory, which means they have to deal with each invader as if it was seen for the first time. However, NK cells are responsive to the cytokines: interleukin-3 and interleukin-4. IL-4 stimulates NK function, while IL-3 prevents their death.[5]

Natural killer cells have some properties similar to cytotoxic T cells, which kill cell invaders by releasing toxic enzymes. NK cells, however, are more voracious killers than cytotoxic T cells. NK cells provide the first line of attack against cancer cells and cells infected by pathogens other than viruses. Research shows that cancer patients have a reduced number of NK cells, and the reduction is associated with the severity of the cancer.

NK cells do not need "permission" from the T_4 cell (helper T cell) and are free to attack. Of particular interest is the ability of NK cells to release interferons, proteins that stop viruses from replicating. These interferons also improve the killing ability of NK cells, making them more aggressive and calling more NK cells to arms.

Cytotoxic T Cells

Cytotoxic T cells, also called killer T cells, travel to the site of invasion, where they attach to malignant cells or infected cells. Cytotoxic T cells also have specialized surface receptors that can recognize specific antigens. They also release a messenger that improves the eating and digesting activity of macrophages, attracts more macrophages to the site, and encourages the macrophages to stay at the site of infection. Most important, cytotoxic T cells also secrete interferons, which stop viruses from reproducing and enhance the killing action of the T cells themselves. Cytotoxic T cells are especially effective against cancer cells and slow-growing bacteria, such as tuberculosis.

Suppressor T Cells

Suppressor T cells shut down certain activities of the immune response several weeks after an infection. They help maintain a balance in the immune system until another microbial threat arrives. Suppressor T cells also stop cytotoxic T cells from releasing chemicals and producing antibodies. A normal ratio of helper T cells to suppressor T cells is 2:1. When suppressor cells are reduced, B cells are left to continue their function, unregulated, wreaking havoc on the body.

Interferons

Interferons are the immune system's front-line defense against most viruses. Several types of interferons exist—gamma, beta, and alpha interferon. Interferons beef up noninfected cells' resistance to viral infections. Viruses can only cause disease if they can duplicate themselves within cells. Interferons are potent virus killers because they halt that replication process. Interferon is also secreted by T cells in order to call NK cells to battle at the site of infected cells. Although the U.S. Food and Drug Administration (FDA) has approved a synthesized interferon for application in various human diseases, results have been disappointing and side effects severe.

B Cells

The body not only produces millions of T cells but also millions of B cells, all of which are capable of responding to their own specific antigens. B cells derive mainly from bone marrow and set up house in the lymph nodes; unlike T cells, they do not circulate in the blood. Their role is to produce and secrete antibodies. Each B cell is specific to one particular antigen. B cells ensure antibody production against antigens with the help of T cells. They signal that an antigen is present in order for a T cell to do its work.

When an invader is present, T cells tell B cells to start producing antibodies. B cells then turn into plasma cells, whereby millions of antibodies specific to the invaded cells are produced. Once the antibodies are produced, they are sent into the bloodstream to lock onto an antigen and destroy it. Many antibodies may coat an invader, often completely inactivating it or halting it long enough to mark it for destruction by other immune cells. Plasma cells memorize the invader's antigens and become memory B cells. In this way, if another invasion occurs, antibodies will be made available much more rapidly. Plasma cells are relatively short-lived, lasting only four to five days. During this time, antibodies are secreted at a rapid rate. The B cells that do not become plasma cells remain as memory B cells and live for months or years, ready to take rapid action the next time the same invader appears. Memory cells, like elephants, never forget.

Antibodies

Antibodies are the body's infection fighters. The five classes of antibodies called immunoglobulin (Ig) include IgA, IgE, and IgM.

IgA is found in tears, milk, sweat, and saliva, as well as on mucous membranes. It either holds off invaders or pushes them out of the body. When secretory IgA (found in the gastrointestinal tract) is low, immune deficiency is common.

IgE is involved in allergic reactions; it encourages cells to release histamine (a substance that mediates allergic reactions). In cases of severe allergic reactions, too much histamine causes a system overload that may result in anaphylactic reactions that can result in death. IgE's protective mechanism triggers inflammatory reactions, which help to protect the body against parasitic infections. The most common types of allergic responses occur when the immune system develops a sensitivity to normally harmless materials such as grass pollens or house dust. The attack against these substances, mediated by IgE, is essentially the same, though more limited than that mounted against viruses and bacteria producing some of the same symptoms.

Like other antibodies, each IgE is specific for a particular antigen. Highly allergic animals may suffer a multitude of symptoms—not due to a hyperactive immune system, as some believe—but due to a severely compromised and unbalanced immune system. Steroids and antihistamines only treat the symptoms and not the root cause of a weakened immune system.

IgG is the most abundant antibody. It coats microbes and is specialized to kill certain abundant bacteria and viruses. It also activates a series of enzymes that enhance the digestion of invaders. IgG can punch holes in cell membranes, allowing access to the internal contents of the cell, which is especially important for attacking intracellular viruses.

Because of their large size, IgM molecules are usually confined to the bloodstream and are, therefore, probably of little importance in conferring protection in tissues.

Helper T Cells

There are two types of T helper cells: the so-called TH_1 (CD4) cells and the TH_2 (CD4) cells. TH_1 cells produce IL-2 (interleukin-2) and gamma interferon (IFN-g), and the TH_2 cells release IL-4, IL-6, IL-10, which enhance the activity of B cells to produce antibodies.

Many chronic diseases occur when TH_1 cell activity is either defective or suppressed, and there is an overactivity of antibody production. On the other hand, the CD8 (cytotoxic) positive cells are activated by the TH_1 lymphokines to become killer cells, which destroy the host cells harboring the pathogen (intracellular). This is an escape route utilized by certain organisms in an attempt to evade the initial response mounted by the antibodies produced by B cells. This is due to the fact that once inside the host cell, the pathogens are inaccessible to the action of antibodies. Cytotoxic T cells must be activated by TH_1 cells to do their job. Therefore, TH_1 cells produce lymphokines that enhance the ability of the immune system to respond to viruses, intracellular bacteria, fungi, or parasites; they also activate cytotoxic or suppressor T cells. These cells rush out and destroy abnormal cells infected with bacteria, viruses, and cancer. TH_1 cells also control the activity of TH_2 cells.

In general, TH_1 cells stimulate cellular immunity and down regulate TH_2 cells, which stimulate humoral immunity, eosinophil, and mast cells.[6] It is interesting to note that most diseases typically involve either TH_1 or TH_2 responses.

Bacteria and viruses usually initiate a TH_1 response, which promotes an immune reaction that destroys the infection. Some infectious diseases (for example, feline immunodeficiency virus or FIV as it is commonly called) initiate a TH_1 response, but if the infection is not completely cleared, the immune reaction may switch to the TH_2 response. When the TH_2 response becomes the predominant reaction in an infection, various pathological processes such as allergies, atopic dermatitis, autoimmune diseases, asthma, and inflammatory bowel disease occur. The TH_1 response may be an adaptation by the body to prevent damaging immune responses by TH_2 cells in chronic diseases. Remember TH_1 cells down regulate TH_2 cells.

Humans and animals with atopic dermatitis seem to have a proliferation of TH_2 cells. Allergies of any kind are an abnormal immunologic condition associated with an exaggerated TH_2 response. It is important to note that in vitro studies in mice suggest that glucocorticoids may promote TH_2 cell proliferation.[7] Atopic dermatitis is frequently treated with steroids; however, if glucocorticoids promote the response that they are used to suppress, then such treatment could be harmful in the long run. This is proof that steroids are not the answer. The more severe the inflammatory reactions, the larger the disparity between TH_1 and TH_2 cells. Allergies are an imbalance between TH_1 and TH_2 cells in which the TH_1 cells are deficient and the TH_2 cells are prolific. With chronic diseases involving the TH_2 response that leads to systemic disease, modulating and enhancing the immune system will lead to switching to the protective TH_1 subset and resolution of the disease.[8] We will discuss treatment options later in this chapter.

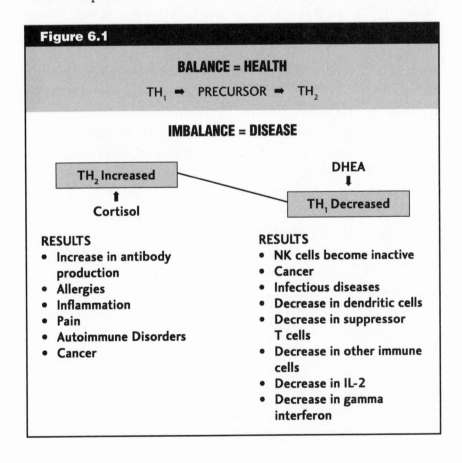

Figure 6.1

BALANCE = HEALTH

TH_1 ➡ PRECURSOR ➡ TH_2

IMBALANCE = DISEASE

TH₂ Increased

↑
Cortisol

DHEA
↓
TH₁ Decreased

RESULTS
• Increase in antibody production
• Allergies
• Inflammation
• Pain
• Autoimmune Disorders
• Cancer

RESULTS
• NK cells become inactive
• Cancer
• Infectious diseases
• Decrease in dendritic cells
• Decrease in suppressor T cells
• Decrease in other immune cells
• Decrease in IL-2
• Decrease in gamma interferon

INTERLEUKINS

Interleukins are cytokines (proteins that alert the body to mount a defense). They regulate the interactions between leukocytes.

Interleukin-1

Interleukin-1 (IL-1) is involved in the process that induces fever, which helps in the destruction of a virus or bacteria. Macrophages produce the most IL-1. Once IL-1 is released, it encourages T cells to produce more interleukin-2. IL-1 is an essential initiating factor for the immune and inflammatory responses.

Interleukin-2

Interleukin-2 (IL-2) helps helper T cells to tell cytotoxic T cells to destroy an invader. It also informs all T cells to release more IL-2 as required and, therefore, be able to destroy more invaders. It is especially effective in enhancing immune responses against tumors. Interleukin-2 is a powerful immunomodulator, which also causes more T cells to be produced.

Interleukin-3

Interleukin-3 (IL-3) promotes the growth and maturation of bone marrow stem cells. Its main function is to recruit eosinophils, neutrophils, and monocytes. It also stimulates B cells to secrete immunoglobulins.

Interleukin-4

Interleukin-4 (IL-4) enhances the ability of B cells to make antibodies (IgG and IgE). It also stimulates helper T cells and cytotoxic T cells to perform their job. Overproduction of IL-4 promotes allergic responses.

Interleukin-5

Interleukin-5 (IL-5) increases the proliferation of activated B cells. It stimulates IgG, IgA, and IgM production and enhances IL-4 induced IgE production. IL-5 stimulates eosinophil function, which plays a role in allergic reactions.

Interleukin-6
Interleukin-6 (IL-6) is released by macrophages, monocytes, and some T cells; it also induces B cells to produce antibodies. Abnormal production of IL-6 is associated with autoimmune disorders and inflammatory and allergic conditions. Studies show that psoriasis is associated with TH_2 cells releasing an overabundance of IL-6, which increases the production of skin cells.[9] IL-6, like IL-1, plays an important role in systemic inflammatory response. It is found in high concentrations in the ascitic fluid in cats suffering from feline infectious peritonitis.[10]

Interleukin-7
Interleukin-7 (IL-7) induces proliferation of pre-B cells, thymocytes, and T cells. It stimulates CD4+ and CD8+ cells and induces the expression of IL-2. IL-7 is an essential player in cell-mediated immunity and has a normalizing affect on the immune system.

Interleukin-8
Neutrophils release large amounts of interleukin-8 (IL-8) during phagoctyosis. It is a chemotactic (messenger) agent to T cells, neutrophils, and basophils.

Interleukin-9
Interleukin-9 (IL-9) enhances the proliferation response of mast cells to IL-3.

Interleukin-10
Interleukin-10 (IL-10) is a protein secreted by some B cell lymphomas and by helper T cell clones in response to antigens. It also inhibits cytokines such as IL-2 or gamma interferon, which are associated with TH_1 subsets.

Interleukin-11
Interleukin-11 (IL-11) stimulates certain B cells and is associated with IL-6 and IL-3 to enhance antibody production.

Interleukin-12
Interleukin-12 (IL-12) enhances the cytotoxic effects of T cells and natural killer cells. It also induces gamma interferon and IL-2 production and proliferation.

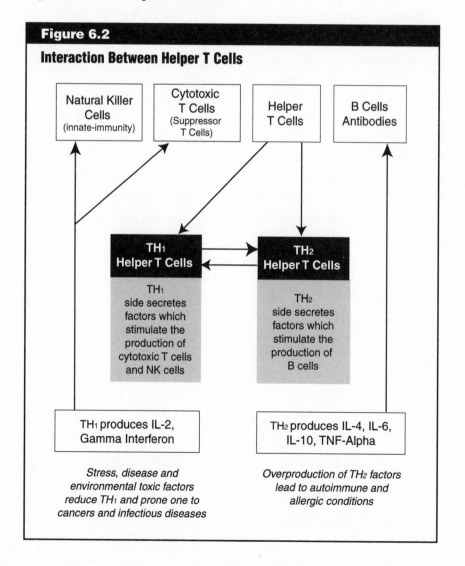

Figure 6.2

Interaction Between Helper T Cells

BIOLOGICAL RESPONSE MODIFIERS

Biological response modifiers (BRMs) are substances that down regulate when the immune system is hyperactive and up regulate when the immune system is suppressed. In short, with most diseases, the immune system is unbalanced and therefore biological response modifiers rebalance the immune system. Given the correct tools, the body will shift toward balance and health.

A common denominator among immunomodulating herbs (BRMs) is the presence of complex sugar molecules known as polysaccharides. Polysaccharides improve the activity of lymphocytes and other cells of the immune system, thus strengthening the overall immune response.[11]

Plant polysaccharides—and particularly mushroom polysaccharides—are frequently described as immune-enhancing agents. I've used a number of them successfully for a variety of diseases, including cancers. Clinical trials conducted in Japan with two polysaccharide products approved by the Ministry of Health indicate significant benefits to human cancer patients when these products are used as adjuvants to standard medical therapies.[12]

Polysaccharides are natural products that consist of numerous sugar molecules linked together to form complex chains. Most of the sugar molecules in these chains are glucose; some are similar sugars such as galactase, fucose, arabinose, xylose, rhamnose, and mannose. Polysaccharides form a broad class of natural substances that include some of the most common plant constituents, notably starch and cellulose.

Starch is the form of sugars that plants utilize for storage of energy, which is derived from sunlight and is to be used later for metabolic energy or as a starting material for producing other molecules. Starch is the main natural food source of complex carbohydrates for humans; it is mainly obtained in the form of grain (wheat, corn, rice) and certain vegetables (potatoes).

Cellulose is the structural material of plants. Like starch, it is metabolically inactive; however, unlike starch, it does not serve a storage role, for it is not degraded by the plant later if simple carbohydrates are needed. Cellulose, made entirely of glucose, is the principal fiber in foods. It is found in fruits, vegetables, and grain coats. There are two major groups of cellulose fiber—soluble fiber and insoluble fiber. Soluble fiber, such as fruit pectin, has a soothing effect on the intestinal tract. Insoluble fiber helps form the bulk of the feces, and thus regulates elimination. Both forms of fiber are not absorbed, but are passed through the body.

Starch and cellulose, as well as simple sugars, do not have an immunological effect. We are interested in other polysaccharides that have immunomodulating effects. It is not totally clear how immunologically active polysaccharides function. They may simply be another form of cellulose with a slightly different structure. Most plants, perhaps all plants, have them, but the amounts are quite small. They typically make up less than 1 percent of the dried plant material; by contrast, starch and cellulose often make up more than 20 percent of the dried plant, and can make up as much as 80 percent.

It has been suggested that one of the underlying reasons that certain herbs and mushrooms have long been regarded as being healthful in traditional Chinese and Japanese dietary and herbal practices is partly because of their polysaccharides. In particular, astragalus, Lycium fruit, ganoderma, cordyceps, and shiitake, when consumed in large amounts, may provide enough polysaccharides to yield a medicinal immunological effect. All of these herbs are considered health tonics, and all of them, except shiitake, have other active constituents that may explain their effects when consumed in the form and amount traditionally utilized.

Modern research has identified key structural components of immunomodulating herbs. Work is ongoing, and more will be discovered in the future. However, at this point in time, beta-1,3 and beta-1,6 glucose linkage chains are the most important. In one study, it was reported that while beta-glucans from ganoderma were active in laboratory animals in antitumor tests, alpha-glucans from ganoderma were not.[13] In another study, it was revealed that the active polysaccharides of ganoderma have a backbone chain beta-1,3 linkages with a side chain every twelve sugar molecules along the backbone, connected via a beta-1,6 linkage. It has been proposed that the frequency of branching in polysaccharides from several mushrooms is important to their activity.[14]

I've always regarded herbs as nature's drugs, and as such, respect their usage and power of healing. Let's look at some mechanisms of action that possibly show how these gifts from nature work. Several mechanisms have been found in laboratory animals and in vitro (test tube) studies, and these appear to occur in humans when polysaccharides are administered. It is possible that the immune system interacts with the polysaccharides in the same manner as they do to the cell wall glycoproteins of bacteria and yeasts. The initial step of polysaccharides interaction involves the complement component C_3. B cells then become involved, and antibody production is promoted. The cell-mediated immune response is eventually activated, resulting in natural killer cells attacking the cancer or virally infected cells.

In another study, it was concluded that cordyceps polysaccharides can stimulate the growth and maturation of thymocytes (from thymus gland) and selectively induce the differentiation of thymocytes toward CD4+, thus elevating the proportion of CD4+ T cells in peripheral blood lymphocytes.[15] Immune modulation was also shown when astragalus extract was applied to mononuclear cells taken from human cancer patients with chemotherapy-induced immune suppression.[16] Beta-1,3 glucans have been shown to activate macrophages and cytotoxic T cells. Another study indicates that polyporus (mushroom) was able to restore immune function by the release of cytotoxic factors from macrophages that could kill tumor cells.[17] Though these experiments were performed in a laboratory with mice, it shows much promise for dogs, cats, and humans. It was also shown that polysaccharides from tremella mushroom protected bone marrow suppression from cyclophosphamide, an immune suppressive cancer drug. In Japan, extensive research has been done on PSK derived from coriolus mushroom and is readily used as an adjunct in cancer patients. When the blood of cancer patients given PSK was analyzed, leukocyte levels, macrophages, killer cell activity, T cell profiles, and other parameters indicated immune enhancement.[18]

A vast amount of research effort has been devoted to immunologically active polysaccharides. The combination of chemical tests, laboratory testing, and clinical testing leads one to believe that there is a value in applying these polysaccharides in immune compromised animals that are experiencing allergies, chronic infections, autoimmune diseases, and cancers. Unfortunately, the herb industry is unregulated, and with all the popularity of herbs these days, what is bought and sold at health food stores is mostly useless material.

Astragalus

Astragalus is becoming a popular immune stimulant in the U.S., as evidence of its effect on the immune system continues to accumulate. Research to date shows that this remarkable plant stimulates the immune system in many ways. This modern research validates some ancient uses of the plant in China, where it has been used for thousands of years.

Astragalus, like many other toxic herbs used in China, contains triterpenoid saponins. These compounds are analogous to the steroid hormones of the animal world. They have a steroid-like molecule attached to one or more sugar groups.[19] Similar types of triterpenoid saponins have been found in ginseng. These saponins are known as astragalosides, and so far, eight have been described. Besides the saponin, a polysaccharide known as astragalar is known to have immunological activity.

This herb is one of the classical and most important in the arsenal of Oriental tonic and health promoting medicinal plants. Astragalus has been in the limelight in recent years as a possible answer for a range of human diseases. It is probably the most hopeful new natural remedy for human AIDS, viral hepatitis, other viral diseases, myasthenia gravis, and, especially, immune restoration of cancer patients. In cancer patients, it is proposed as a treatment to strengthen the cellular immunity, which has been seriously compromised by the disease and/or by chemotherapy or radiotherapy.

In pharmacological experiments with mice, an astragalus extract was found to dramatically enhance the activity of the immune system (natural killer cells). This may be caused by stimulation of interferon.[20] When an astragalus extract was injected into mice infected with Newcastle Disease virus or Sendai virus, interferon production was increased and the injected mice survived longer than control subjects. Human subjects with cancer, who were injected with an extract of astragalus, also made more interferon.[21]

Studies at the University of Texas's M.D. Anderson Hospital and Tumor Institute found that the T cell function of cancer patients was extremely low (26) compared to normal people (82). When astragalus was added to a test tube containing the T cells of cancer patients, T cell function increased to 113, more than the normal.[22] It was found that the most effective component of astragalus was a polysaccharide, lending support to the use of the whole plant and not any one extract. I always use astragalus for any immune related disorder, especially cancer.

Beta-1,3 D-Glucan

A dietary supplement called beta-1,3 D-glucan is the latest immune-enhancing nutritional supplement to enter the complementary medical arena. While relatively new to the natural foods and alternative medicine industry, beta-1,3 D-glucan has been extensively researched for its immune-enhancing ability.[23] It's not a drug, vitamin, mineral, or herb; rather, it is a natural occurring compound, which is derived from the cell wall of Baker's yeast (Saccharomyces Cerevisiae).

Once the immune system is activated by beta-1,3 D-glucan, the immune system creates a permanent defense against viral, bacterial, fungal, parasitic, or neoplastic assailants. This immune enhancer seems to selectively stimulate the macrophage part of the immune system first. As discussed earlier, a macrophage is a cell common to all living beings and is often referred to by immunologists as the "Pac-Man" of the immune system. Macrophages are huge cells in comparison to infectious organisms and other immune cells. Macrophages are specialized cells and are first in the line of cell-mediated immune defense. Once activated, the macrophages create a chain reaction, which results in mobilizing and amplifying the entire immune system. A special receptor site, specific to beta-1,3 D-glucan, exists on the macrophage. Beta-1,3 D-glucan binds to the receptor site, thereby fully activating the macrophage.

When the beta-1,3 D-glucan activates the macrophage, it enhances "phagoctyosis," which is the ability of the macrophage to engulf and destroy foreign cells. Resembling an octopus, the macrophage extends tentacle-like arms, physically pulling in infectious invaders, ingesting them, and destroying them with powerful enzymes. In addition to ingesting foreign invaders, the macrophage is the first link in intercellular communication with the immune system. This results in the mobilization of the immune system, thus creating a chain reaction. An activated macrophage accomplishes this communication by producing important immune system messengers (IL-1, IL-2, IL-6), interferons, colony stimulating factors, etc. Natural killer cells, B cells, complement cells, and other immune cells—a cascade of immune system messengers— gather momentum with each exchange of signals among macrophages and amplify the immune response until the enemy is defeated. When fully activated, the macrophage becomes a "tank."

In one study, women who had experienced recurrent malignant ulcers of the chest wall following mastectomy and radiation for breast cancer were treated with beta-1,3 D-glucan and completely healed.[24]

Beta-1,3 D-glucan is a safe and potent nutritional supplement with a nonspecific immune stimulation, which also possesses potent free-radical scavenging activity. I have used the supplement for a number of infections, cancers, and even asthma. Technically, it is a polysaccharide molecule made completely with glucose that is highly purified. However, this is different from energy-storing glucose containing polysaccharides because the connection between units is different. It is safe, and I use it in the treatment of all serious maladies.

Colostrum
A newborn's very first meal is of great significance to its health and well-being for the rest of its life. The immune system of the newborn is not fully developed, making it highly susceptible to numerous pathogens, antigens, and allergens. Mother's milk provides individualized nutritional food to promote passive immunity and proper growth and development. Colostrum provided in breast milk contains all the immune factors needed while the newborn's own system develops.

There are numerous constituents in colostrum, and research is identifying new ones at a rapid pace. We will only discuss a few at this time. Colostrum and its immune-boosting properties are by no means limited to humans. In fact, all mammals pass on immunities from mother to offspring. Even more fascinating is the fact that antibodies by one species can actually strengthen the immune system of another species. Tests in which colostrum preparations from cattle were administered to mice showed a positive effect on the immune systems of the test subjects.[25] Research at South Dakota State University demonstrated that by giving colostrum to young animal subjects infected with E. coli, lesions and immunosuppression linked to this bacteria could be inhibited.[26] Other strains of bacteria, though not destroyed by colostrum, were strongly inhibited in their growth. Even more interesting is that friendly bacteria were not destroyed by colostrum. Recently, it has been shown that colostrum contains cytokines and other protein compounds of very low molecular weight so that they can act as biological response modifiers (BRMs), which intervene in biological processes. It has now been clarified that there are at least four cytokines in colostrum: IL-1 followed by IL-2 were discovered to be part of the colostral factors that stimulate resistance to infections. IL-6, tissue necrosis factor (TNF), and gamma interferon are thought to protect the newborn's gastrointestinal tract by stimulating the immune system.

There is evidence of IgE transference by colostrum to calves during the first twelve weeks of life, and this is assumed to generate protection against intestinal parasites. IgG, IgA, and IgM are also present in bovine colostrum showing the ability to protect against various infectious diseases.[27]

Proline-rich-polypeptide (PRP), a polypeptide with known immunomodulating activity, is present in colostrum. PRP acts both in vivo and in vitro (test tube) and is not species specific. PRP stimulates immature thymocytes (cells that develop in the thymus gland) to turn into functionally active T cells, the immune system defenders that attack invading organisms directly.[28] PRP also changes surface markers and functions of cells, thereby acting as an immunoregulator.

Recently, lymphokine hormone-like peptides called "infopeptides," which regulate the immune response, were isolated from colostrum. These infopeptides induce the recipient to produce cytokines, which allow the animal to recuperate or reorient its "immunologic memory" in a response to any inflammatory condition (allergy, autoimmunity).[29] I have been using infopeptides for a variety of inflammatory conditions including asthma and allergies. This works as a true immunomodulator due to its induction of anti-inflammatory cytokine-type activity. I have also used a high quality colostrum product from New Zealand with good success in treating a variety of diseases ranging from infections to allergies. Colostrum is not a miracle substance, but it is an excellent immunomodulator. It is safe to use in dogs and cats of all ages with no side effects. In recent times, it has been popularized in the media press with some overestimated effects. As one attempts to strengthen and modulate the immune system, one should scrutinize these products for efficacy.

Cordyceps

Cordyceps sinensis belongs to a group of fungi that includes such delicacies as truffles and morels. It is found in high altitude from 9,000 to 16,000 feet in the mountains of Tibet and China.[30] This is a unique mushroom in that it parasitizes a cold temperature caterpillar that hibernates just below the frozen ground surface.

I have been using cordyceps for quite some time with wonderful results. I use it in all animals that need immune enhancement and are experiencing cancers as well as liver, kidney, and respiratory problems. The commercial cordyceps is grown usually on rice or other media and has been shown to be just as effective as the wild variety. This is the most versatile of all of the medicinal mushrooms that I use, as we will see in later discussions.

For quite some time, cordyceps was best known in the U.S. for its ability to stimulate the immune system. As previously discussed, the compounds responsible for immune activity are long chain sugars known as polysaccharides. The Sichuan Institute of Traditional Chinese Medicine reported that its researchers had isolated a polysaccharide from cordyceps, which had the effect of activating macrophages. The polysaccharide they isolated also stimulated lymphocytes, a vital group of infection fighting white blood cells produced in lymphoid tissue.[31]

An experiment conducted by Shanghai Medical University showed cordyceps can stimulate T- and B-lymphocyte proliferation and has certain effects on mononuclear phagocytes, T-lymphocytes, B-lymphocytes, and NK cells. It is obviously a wide acting immunomodulator.[32]

Another study in rats with chronic renal failure showed that cordyceps can reduce mortality rate, improve anemia, lower levels of BUN and creatinine, and promote splenic lymphocyte transformation rate and interleukin-2 production.[33]

Researchers at Hunan Medical University refer to cordyceps

as one of the most potent herbal tonics in traditional Chinese medicine. Their findings show that cordyceps activates NK cells in vitro and in animals and has significant antitumor activity. They concluded that cordyceps could be used as an immunopotentiating agent both in the treatment of cancer and in patients with deficient immune systems.[34]

It is well known that patients with autoimmune diseases possess low NK cell activity. I have used this herb as adjunctive therapy in all autoimmune and inflammatory conditions. There are no side effects, and it can be used safely in both dogs and cats.

Coriolus

Coriolus versicolor is a mushroom found in wooded temperate zones in North America, Asia, and Europe. Most of the research and usage has come from Japan. In Japan, it is mainly used as an adjunct to radiation and chemotherapy in a variety of cancers.

Two principle immunologically active extracts have been identified and used. As of this writing, it has not been established which extract is more beneficial. One extract known as PSP, a polysaccharide-peptide consisting of 10 percent peptides and 90 percent polysaccharide, has been shown to enhance natural killer (NK) cell function, lymphocyte proliferation, and IgG and IL-2 concentration in immunosuppressed rats.[35] The other extract is well known as PSK (Krestin), a protein-bound polysaccharide. It has demonstrated benefits through a variety of immune actions in human, animal, and in vitro research. PSK has shown to benefit cancer victims by activating macrophage and T killer cell activity, stimulating lymphocyte counts, and balancing helper/suppressor ratios. Human studies, combining PSK with conventional cancer therapy, showed significantly increased survival rates and periods of remission for a number of cancers.[36] I have used both extracts in dogs and cats for a variety of cancers with no toxicity seen. There have been more than four hundred clinical studies performed in the past twenty years demonstrating that this mushroom benefits the immune system.

Echinacea

There are several species of echinacea (angustifolia, pallida, and purpurea), which have therapeutic benefits. This perennial, known by herbalists as the purple coneflower, is a native to the great plains of the United States. Echinacea was one of the most popular herbs used by the Native American Indians. They used it to treat coughs, colds, sore throats, infections, toothaches, and even snake bites.

The active components that occur in the various echinacea preparations can be divided into three major groups: caffeic acid derivatives, polysaccharide fractions, and lipophilic components. Both lipophilic components and caffeic acid derivatives have been shown to stimulate phagoctyosis by macrophages.[37] The polysaccharide fraction has not been shown to have any immune-stimulating effect at this time.

I have used echinacea to treat a variety of diseases for long periods of time with no side effects seen. There has been much confusion as to when and how long to use echinacea. There is no rationale for the limited use of echinacea. The eclectic physicians, a group of nineteenth century physicians, used echinacea for such diseases as abscesses, bee stings, cancer, viral infections, malaria, emphysema, fevers, septic injuries, tuberculosis, tetanus, and more.[38]

Modern research demonstrates that while echinacea was given to patients, phagocytic activity by macrophages remained high. When echinacea was stopped, phagocytic activity remained high for a few days before returning to normal.[39] There was no depletion of activity of macrophages. The concept that the immune system would be depleted with prolonged usage is not supported by modern research.

The immune system is incredibly complex, and an herb such as echinacea, which acts by stimulating phagocytic activity by macrophages, may be beneficial in cancers and even autoimmune conditions. Phagocytic cells are part of nonspecific immunity. These macrophages are a key element in immune surveillance. The macrophages process antigenic material (virus, bacteria, fungus, pollens, parasites, etc.) and then present this to the helper T cells. At this point, the helper T cells join the party and get to work. So, if an herb such as echinacea significantly increases phagocytic activity, the end result will be enhanced immune surveillance.

Echinacea is, in reality, an immunomodulator and not an immunostimulant. If an autoimmune disease is caused by a virus or a bacteria such as tuberculosis, and if they are cleared from the body by the macrophages, then inflammation will decrease. In this way, echinacea can "down regulate" an overactive or an unbalanced immune system. So the body's response to an allergen may be reduced if phagocytic activity by macrophages are enhanced. Remember, the longer echinacea is used, the more prolonged the phagocytic activity is seen.

Ginseng

Ginseng and ginseng products are increasing in popularity. They have been highly valued for thousands of years in many different cultures for their medicinal properties. Ginseng is probably the most highly regarded tonic and adaptogenic herb in the world. There are many different varieties of the ginseng plant grown throughout the world that are used for traditional Chinese medicine. All of the most common species of plants known as ginseng have similar reactions in humans or animals. Ginseng is often used to maintain and support health as a tonic rather than treating a particular disease in the body. However, I have used it successfully in the treatment of a variety of diseases such as immune suppression, cancer, allergies, Addison's disease, respiratory diseases, diabetes, and general weakness. Many older animals especially benefit from its use.

Nearly all ginseng researchers claim that ginseng's reported actions are attributed to the combined effect of its glycoside components called ginsenosides. These components have a structure similar to steroid hormones; however, they do not have a direct hormonal action. Rather, they influence the production of hormones and have other effects.[40] There are at least thirteen different ginsenosides present in Panax ginseng, which are believed to be the most important active constituents.

I believe that when using Panax ginseng, it is important to use it as a complete herb with all of its ginsenosides and not concentrated to any particular ginsenoside. It was found that if the ginsenosides are isolated individually and tested in laboratory animals that each has a somewhat different and sometimes opposite effect.[41] Some attribute the balancing action of ginseng to the complex interaction of different glycoside effects. Thus, to get the desired balancing action of ginseng, it is necessary to utilize the complete set of glycosides rather than isolated ones. I have used standardized extract and found that a crude extract of ginseng had a much better effect.

The immunomodulating effects of Panax ginseng is rarely ever discussed due to its popularity as an adaptogenic tonic. However, almost every immune dysregulated patient I see is put on ginseng. The exceptions are patients with known high blood pressure. Studies have shown that ginseng can increase cell-mediated immunity, natural killer cell activity, interferon production, lymphocyte activation, reticulo-endothelial system proliferation, and phagocytic function.[42] The reticulo-endothelial cells (RES) are the immune system components that devour foreign organisms without leaving their original sites in the liver, spleen, and other tissues of the body.

Glutathione
Glutathione is a sulfur-containing antioxidant composed of glutamic acid, cysteine, and glycine. In the body, glutathione exists in both reduced states (active) and oxidized states (inactive), but all of the vital functions of glutathione are carried out in the reduced states.

Aging, malnutrition, and exposure to toxins diminish blood levels of glutathione. Research demonstrates that low levels of glutathione increase the risk of illnesses such as arthritis, diabetes, cancer, and heart disease.[43] In humans, decreased intracellular levels of glutathione are also associated with peripheral neuropathies, Parkinson's disease, myopathies, hemolytic enemia, pulmonary fibrosis, and decreased helper T cell function.[44-47]

White blood cells attack pathogens such as viruses and unwanted bacteria and disable these dangerous intruders by oxidizing them (chemical warfare). In the process, many free radicals are created. If left unchecked, free radicals can destroy much more than the intruders. These chemicals can destroy the white blood cells themselves. This is how glutathione makes its dramatic contribution—it mops up these free radicals, and so prevents the self-destruction of hardworking white blood cells. In fact, glutathione's work allows white blood cells to increase in numbers and strength.

Two other modes of action might also be significant: Glutathione seems to protect other antioxidants (among them, vitamins C and E) from oxidizing, thereby prolonging and enhancing their effectiveness. It also acts directly against certain carcinogenic substances (alfatoxin B_1) by binding to these toxins and eliminating them through urine or bile.[48]

Raising glutathione levels has been shown to alter the cytokine balance in favor of a TH_1 immune response (anti-inflammatory, anticancer, antiviral), which lowers the TH_2 response (inflammatory).[49]

Now that we know that glutathione is important to maintain optimum health and the prevention of disease, how do we increase it in our pets and ourselves? There are several good natural sources. Most glutathione supplements when ingested are destroyed by the GI tract. I use a stabilized glutathione supplement that is combined with anthocyanins. Anthocyanins are naturally occurring members of the bioflavonoid family; they form the dark red to purple and blue-black pigments found within certain plants such as bilberry. Research has shown that certain antioxidants, such as plant anthocyanins, help maintain adequate intracellular levels of glutathione by recycling oxidized glutathione.[50] It was further shown in animal studies that oral stabilized glutathione administration resulted in a doubling of plasma glutathione levels.[51] It was also absorbed intact into isolated kidney cells via a sodium-dependent pathway. The increase in intracellular reduced glutathione levels protected kidney cells from damage by toxins.[52] I routinely use glutathione in cats with kidney degeneration.

Other good sources of glutathione precursors are raw eggs, raw milk, and whey. There are several companies that claim their whey protein concentrate is the best in increasing glutathione levels. More independent research on their products is needed in order to be accepted. Raw eggs from cage-free chickens are another great source. High levels of glutathione is found in egg whites, so give the whole egg. Don't worry about biotin deficiency unless you feed twenty eggs daily. My cats eat raw eggs daily without any problems. Another great source of glutathione (if you are fortunate to live in a state where it is obtainable) is certified raw milk. I live in California where certified raw milk is available. I personally drink at least a quart daily and make sure that my cats get it daily, too. Raw milk is also high in omega-3 fatty acids; vitamins A, E, and D; taurine (critical for cats); wulzen factor (anti-stiffness factor); and a host of minerals. Raw certified milk is highly palatable for both dogs and cats and is practically a perfect food. If you are unable to obtain it in your state due to archaic laws, write to your legislature. However, it may be obtained directly from a dairy farmer.

Some people have tried to raise glutathione levels by supplementation with N-acetyl cysteine; however, it has been shown to fail in increasing glutathione levels.[53] I have not found it to be of any benefit when taken orally.

Larch Arabinogalactan
Larch arabinogalactan is a polysaccharide derived from the western larch tree. The arabinogalactan is a class of polysaccharide that is also found in a wide range of plants such as leak seeds,

carrots, radishes, sorghum, bamboo grass, and more.[54] A well-known popular herb that many people use, echinacea, contains significant amounts of arabinogalactan.

Much research is being conducted on this herb. Of greatest interest, so far, is how it modulates the immune system. It turns out that arabinogalactan enhances natural killer (NK) cell activity by first increasing interferon gamma (IFN gamma) and other cytokines within the immune system armamentarium.[55]

Two other attributes of larch arabinogalactan make it a versatile herb that may be used in the treatment of many diseases. Arabinogalactan is a source of dietary fiber, which has been shown to increase the production of short-chain fatty acids, which in turn decreases the generation and absorption of ammonia.[56] This attribute may have values in the treatment of porto-systemic encephalopathy because of the ability to lower ammonia in the gastrointestinal tract.

Larch arabinogalactan has also been shown to have a potential as an antimetastatic agent, especially of the liver.[57] I use it in most cases of malignant tumors. It is a fine white powder with a slightly bitter taste. Most dogs, however, will accept it readily in food.

Maitake

For more than 3,000 years, Traditional Chinese Medicine (TCM) has enjoyed an illustrious history. Today, TCM and western medicine function side by side in Japan, as can be witnessed by the frequent use of maitake and other mushrooms to deal with conditions, which, in the U.S., are usually treated with drugs. In Japan, maitake mushrooms are highly prized both as food and medicine. However, until recently, western medicine has never viewed mushrooms as a treatment option for illness or disease. In the 1990s, however, the mushroom received increased clinical and research attention.[58]

Some researchers believe that maitake is the most powerful of all the medicinal mushrooms. I use at least a half dozen medicinal mushrooms, and research is constantly discovering new ones. At this point, I have not ascertained which mushroom is the most medicinally active. If I have, I would have certainly only used that one. So, at Highlands Vet Hospital, I use many different herbs because no herb has "magical" powers and what works in one patient for one disease may not work in another. All of my patients get the benefits of the latest in both western and complementary therapies.

Many researchers believe that maitake's antitumor activity is due to the effect its polysaccharide fraction has on the immune system. Chemically, maitake contains powerful active polysaccharides, especially the immunoenhancing beta D-glucans. Recently, studies have shown that the so-called D-fraction extracted and purified from the fruit body (mushroom) of maitake provides important therapeutic benefits including immunostimulation and tumor inhibition.[59] According to Dr. H. Nanba, who has researched maitake extensively, D-fraction provides immune actions by:

1. Activating cellular immunity.

2. Protecting normal cells from carcinogens.

3. Inhibiting tumor growth.

4. Preventing tumor metastasis.

5. Alleviating the side effects of chemotherapy.

Nanba found that the activity of natural killer cells, cytotoxic T cells, and delayed-hypersensitive T cells were all increased by maitake D-fraction. Also, it was observed that production of interleukin-1 (which activates T cells) and super-oxide anion (which damages tumor cells) was enhanced. The production of interleukin-2 (which activates cytotoxic T cells) was also observed to increase.

Further research by Nanba shows that maitake may even help prevent destruction of T helper cells by HIV virus in humans by as much as 99 percent.[60]

I have used maitake D-fraction for a number of years in both dogs and cats as an adjunct for a number of immune-debilitating diseases, including cancers. I use capsules in dogs and a palatable liquid extract in cats.

Reishi

This mushroom has been cherished in China and Japan for more than two thousand years. Reishi has had quite a reputation in the treatment of such ailments as hepatitis, hypertension, arthritis, allergies, bronchitis, asthma, ulcers, and cancers.[61] In the Orient, few plants are so highly regarded and, to this day, reishi is taken as a longevity herb to preserve youth and health.

Reishi is a true adaptagen, enhancing health and normal functions of the body. For example, while it increases some components of the immune response to cancers, it also inhibits pathological immune functions in autoimmune diseases. It has also been reported to reduce the histamine release associated with allergic reactions, and even to help prevent life threatening anaphylactic reactions.[62]

As with other mushrooms, reishi is nutritionally rich. Among its key ingredients are carbohydrates (sugars and polysaccharides) and proteins with all the essential and nonessential amino acids. The fatty acids in reishi are primarily oleic acid, an unsaturated fatty acid. It contains vitamins B_2, B_3, B_5, C, and D as well as minerals. Other important active ingredients include ganoderic acids, which are steroid-like in structure and provide anti-allergy benefits. Two other key ingredients include polysaccharides and ergosterols, which work together to stimulate natural immune functions.[63]

Research in Japan indicates that the beneficial effects of reishi may be enhanced by the ingestion of vitamin C. It is believed that vitamin C reduces the high molecular weight of the polyaccharides. As the vitamin breaks up these sugars, their viscosity drops and their bio-availability increases. This may also be true of other medicinal mushrooms.[64] Once the polysaccharides are reduced, it is believed, they are more accessible to the immune system cell called the macrophage. Remember, these are nonspecific "Pac Man"-like immune cells that literally gobble up invaders. When the macrophage becomes activated, it signals helper T cells to get to work. From research in China and Japan, the immune cells being activated by reishi to kill tumor cells are primarily the macrophages and helper T cells.[65] I have used reishi either alone or in combination with other medicinal mushrooms for years. I have had great success with its immunomodulating ability. I have used it in the treatment of such diseases as cancer, allergies, chronic infections, asthma, and generalized weakness. One of the most interesting aspects of this herb is that it allows the body to assimilate more oxygen. A study in China for altitude sickness found that it prevented the symptoms in 97.5 percent of 238 soldiers. In the control group, 80.31 percent experienced altitude sickness.[66] This may be a reason I've seen debilitated pets heal quickly. Reishi is a good adjunct to most chronic diseases and is quite safe.

Shiitake

Shiitake has been a prized mushroom in China and Japan for thousands of years. This therapeutic food is now also gaining popularity in the U.S. and is found in most grocery stores. Shiitake is packed with nutrients, which contribute to its therapeutic effects. Scientific analysis has found that shiitake contains vitamins (including B_1, B_2, B_{12}, C, and D), niacin, and pantothenic acid. It is also rich in various minerals. It is believed that the cap of the mushroom has a higher concentration of nutrients than the stem.[67]

Shiitake's principle therapeutic components are composed of Lentinula Edodes Mycelim extract (LEM) and lentinan. It is not important which part of the mushroom these polysaccharides are derived from; however, their pharmacological qualities are interesting. These substances work by enhancing various immune system functions and thus have indirect antiviral and antitumor effects. Lentinan has been shown to activate natural killer cells in both humans and animals, as well as to induce proliferation of peripheral mononuclear cells (PMN).[68, 69] In Japan, where lentinan is available for intravenous injections, it has been shown to significantly increase blood mononuclear cells, IL-1, and tumor necrosis factor (TNF-a).[71] There are other immune parameters that have been shown to benefit humans and animals as well. What is important is that this herb is readily available and safe. I have been using shiitake for many years with promising results. I usually use the medicinal mushrooms together, as I believe there are synergistic effects at work. High quality standardized medicinal mushrooms are available and should be used at all times. There are certainly other medicinal mushrooms in the marketplace, but I wanted to expose the reader to a few of the more popular ones and those proven effective by extensive research. No doubt in the future there will be other mushrooms to benefit the health of humans and animals.

Sterols/Sterolins

Plant sterols and sterolins are among the many phytochemicals, which have in recent years stimulated research into the healing and curing effects of plants against disease. Most of the research on this comes from South Africa.[71] They are plant fats present in every plant (fruits and vegetables), and although chemically similar to the animal fat, cholesterol, they are totally different in biological functions. In the natural state, sterols/sterolins are bound to the fibers of the plant. Thus, they may make it more difficult to digest and absorb during normal digestion.

Seeds and sprouts are the richest sources of sterols/sterolins. However, the refining processes applied in the food industry render the foods useless because they remove the sterols and sterolins to make the products more appealing to the eye (removing precipitation in the extraction of oils from seeds).

Sterols/sterolins have been shown to modulate the functions of the T cells both in patients and in vitro (test tube) by enhancing their cellular division and secretions of lymphokines (IL-2 and gamma interferon). Research has shown that the ingestion of sterols/sterolins is selective in that the TH_1 cells seem to be enhanced, leaving the activity of the TH_2 helper cells unaffected. As discussed earlier, these specific lymphokines are responsible for controlling the activity of B cells. Both IL-2 and gamma interferon are able to switch off the release of the lymphokines, which help the B cells to make antibodies, and thus decreasing the inflammatory response without inhibiting the viral, bacterial, or cancer killing ability.[72] Remember, the immune system is finely tuned to adapt to changes, which can be induced either when a virus or bacterium invades the host or to recognize cancer cells. It therefore stands to reason that when the TH_1 subset of the T cells is deficient, the end result is infection, chronic inflammation, and eventually tissue damage and disease.

In the case of an autoimmune disease, it is thought that the overactivity of the B cells is directly involved in the release of antibodies, which attack the body and cause inflammation. Furthermore, it has been shown that the synthesis and release of IL-6 and tumor necrosis factor (pro-inflammatory) are switched off when macrophages are cultured in the presence of sterols and sterolins.[73] These plant fats seem to help cases of chronic inflammation and are quite safe. I have been using them for more than two years with encouraging results in the treatment of a number of inflammatory and infectious diseases.

As can be imagined, sterols/sterolins research is ongoing as an adjunct treatment for human AIDS patients. Domestic cats with the retro virus feline immunodeficiency virus (FIV), which were given sterols/sterolins, were shown to have 20 percent mortality, while the placebo group had 75 percent mortality after three years. Although the sterols/sterolins have no antiviral activity, the immunomodulatory activity of IL-6 levels leads indirectly to lower viral load levels.[74]

The sterols/sterolins complex is a new natural immune modulator, which has demonstrated promising results in a number of clinical trials.[75, 76] These plant constituents seem to specifically target T helper cells and may help restore balance between TH_1

and TH_2 cells. The end result of this immune modulation is an increase in TH_1 related cytokines, a decrease in TH_2 related cytokines, increased lymphocyte proliferation, and greater natural killer cell activity. This has great potential in treating such diseases as arthritis, allergies, infections, autoimmune diseases, and cancers. Though I have used sterols/sterolins with other herbs, I've been encouraged by the results I've seen in many diseases.

Thymus Extract

For hundreds of years, people have believed that "like heals like." So, someone with liver or heart problems would take beef liver or tissue from beef heart, or someone with immune dysfunction would ingest the thymus gland. Fortunately, these cell tissues are not species-specific, which means bovine extracts are readily accepted by nonrelated species.

Studies indicate that tissue extracted from endocrine glands (glands that secrete hormones) is rich in active hormones, enzymes, proteins, vitamins, and minerals, and that when consumed, many of these compounds can be absorbed intact with great health benefits. These glands include the thyroid, adrenals, pituitary, thymus, and gonads.[77]

The thymus is the major gland of the immune system. It is composed of two soft pinkish-gray lobes and is located above the heart; it appears as a "sail" on x-rays of young animals. For the most part, the health of the thymus determines the health of the immune system. Humans who get frequent infections or suffer from chronic infections or colds must have impaired thymus activity. Also, animals affected with chronic allergies, bacterial infections, autoimmune diseases, and even cancers usually have altered thymus function.

The thymus gland is responsible for many immune system functions, including the production of T-lymphocytes (cell-mediated immunity). These cells do not produce antibodies. It is extremely important in the resistance to infection by bacteria, fungi, yeast, viruses, and various parasites. If an individual suffers from any of these chronic infections, usually his or her cell-mediated immunity is not functioning well.

Like other endocrine organs, the thymus releases hormones. These hormones, which are vitally important because they regulate many immune functions, are thymosin, thymopoetin, and serum thymic factor. Low levels of these hormones in the blood are associated with depressed immunity and an increased susceptibility to infection. Unfortunately, as animals and humans age, the thymus gland involutes and fewer hormones are produced, which makes the body more vulnerable to serious diseases including cancers.

The good news is that there are ways of promoting optimal thymus gland activity. The most basic way is by eating a good natural raw/unprocessed diet. All nutrients should be in their natural state as nature intended, and synthetic so-called vitamins and mineral supplements should be avoided. For example, raw meat and raw unprocessed milk (if accessible) are high in natural vitamins E and A, fatty acids, vitC, selenium, zinc, enzymes, and other nutrients. Raw milk is nearly perfect food and is part of my—and my cats'—daily diet. Unfortunately, it is not available in many states.

Orally administered thymus extracts have been shown to bolster the thymus gland. Many researchers believe that predigested calf thymus extract, which is rich in thymus-derived polypeptides, is effective in correcting many immune derangements.[78, 79] Double-blind studies in children revealed that orally administered thymus extracts are not only able to effectively eliminate infection, but that treatment over a course of a year reduces the number of respiratory infections and significantly improves numerous immune parameter.[80]

I routinely use a thymus extract in allergies and autoimmune diseases with good results. There have been double-blind studies showing that oral administration of thymus extracts can improve the symptoms of hay fever, allergic rhinitis, eczema, food allergies, and autoimmune disease.[81, 82, 83] Clinical improvement is caused by reduced levels of IgE and eosinophils while normalizing the T helper-to-suppressor cell ratios.

Uncaria Tomentosa (Cat's Claw)

In recent years, there has been considerable medical interest in the bark, root, and leaves of a vine found in Peru, Columbia, Ecuador, and other Latin American countries. Called Cat's Claw, this natural product has been hailed, in anecdotes, as the "wonder drug" of the botanical kingdom. Cat's Claw is composed of numerous alkaloids, nonalkaloid glycosides, sterols, and antioxidants.[84] To date, research has identified more than fifty alkaloids in Cat's Claw, with some having therapeutic effects.[85]

In the United States, there are more than fifty different Cat's Claw products. However, most have little or no therapeutic effects. I have used numerous Cat's Claw products from different companies touting how their product is the best on the marketplace—with disappointing results. The main problem stems from the fact that many of these products had little or no therapeutic compounds in their capsules. Recently, I have used a product imported from Austria that has great therapeutic effects. This Cat's Claw known as Seventaro® is high in pentacyclic alkaloids known for their immune-activating effects.[86]

In traditional Peruvian medicine, Uncaria tomentosa has been used for a variety of ailments including abscesses, arthritis, asthma, cancer, fever, ulcers, inflammation, wounds, etc. Klaus Keplinger in Austria has been doing research on the various alkaloids in Cat's Claw for more than twenty-five years. His research shows that if a Cat's Claw root is high in pentacyclic alkaloids and low in tetracyclic alkaloids, it will be much more active on the immune system than a root that is high in tetracyclic alkaloids. That is because the pentacyclic alkaloids are compounds that appear to be responsible for the integrity of the beneficial effects of Cat's Claw on the immune system. The tetracyclic alkaloids block the effects of the pentacyclic alkaloids. In this case, it is important to know exactly which alkaloids are standardized. Some companies standardize the wrong constituents, and thus, no therapeutic effects will be observed. Most of the recent scientific research on Cat's Claw has focused on the effects of various pentacyclic alkaloids and other constituents on the immune system. Some of the effects noted with the pentacyclic alkaloids include powerful effects on phagoctyosis and increases in helper T cells. Pentacyclic alkaloids appear to even expedite wound healing.[87]

In 1993, at the 41st Annual Congress on Medicinal Plant Research in Dusseldorf, Germany, researchers from the Department of Internal Medicine at the University of Innsbruck presented a report of their findings with Cat's Claw against leukemia. They tested six pentacyclic alkaloids in Cat's Claw by placing them in cultures with leukemia cells. Their observations showed that these specific alkaloids inhibit the proliferation of leukemia cells.[88]

One of the possible mechanisms of the antileukemic activity may be the inhibition of the DNA polymerase enzyme system (which allows abnormal cells to proliferate). There are no side effects noted, and stem cells in the bone marrow were left unharmed, unlike standard chemotherapy. So, Cat's Claw also appears to have selective antileukemic activity.

Uncaria tomentosa is probably the most versatile herb that I use. I have used the standardized extract from Austria for chronic infections, cancers, allergies, asthma, and other immune derangements.

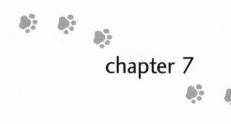

chapter 7

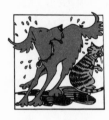

Have Patience When Treating Skin Diseases

Skin diseases in dogs and cats represent a significant caseload in most U.S. veterinary clinics. At times, these are frustrating cases and diagnosis may not be as obvious as it seems at first. Each chronic case should be given a thorough work-up with no stone left unturned. Many diseases have a deeper root, and short-term "quick fixes" with cortisone will only exacerbate the problem. Both the clinician and the pet guardian must be patient; treating the root cause of skin diseases is often a lifelong endeavor.

FLEAS AND TICKS
Both fleas and ticks can carry diseases and certainly can cause much discomfort in both humans and their pets. Modern veterinary medicine has made tremendous strides in controlling these pests. I urge anyone to use modern, proven, and safe treatments available at most veterinary hospitals. Pets get relief quickly and are much happier.

SARCOPTIC MANGE

Sarcoptic mange, or canine scabies, is a commonly encountered parasitic disease of dogs. This microscopic mite may transiently infest humans. It is the most pruritic (causing itching) of all skin diseases and will absolutely not respond to corticosteroid therapy. I usually diagnose it in stray or shelter dogs.

Infested dogs constantly scratch to the point of exhaustion. There is a generalized itching, and lesions or scabs are frequently seen at the ear tips and elbows. The abdomen may appear pink, and there may be areas of lichenification (thickened skin). Multiple skin scraping may reveal a crab-like mite; however, if one has a high degree of suspicion despite negative findings, then treatments should proceed. Diagnosis will be made by response to treatment.

Sarcoptic mange is easily treated by modern western modalities. There are effective dips, and in non-Collie or herding-type breeds, Ivomec works wonderfully. These treatments are safe, and I use them frequently with great success. These dogs suffer, and modern proven treatments bring relief quickly.

DEMODECTIC MANGE

Canine demodectic mange (red mange) is caused by a follicular mite that is a normal inhabitant of the skin. This mite has an elongated appearance and lives in hair follicles and sebaceous glands and is thought to consume epithelial cell secretions.[1] Probably 90 percent of all dogs live in harmony with this mite.

This mite is not contagious, though it is transmitted from the dam to her puppies by direct contact while nursing. Humans have their own demodectic mite with a similar appearance, and under normal conditions, it does not cause pathology.

Two clinical forms of demodicosis are recognized. The most common and benign form is the localized form. This is usually self-limited in young dogs and appears as local patches of alopecia mostly on the face and forelimbs. There is no itching unless it is accompanied by bacterial, fungal, or yeast infections. I always culture these puppies for fungal disease because many are also pruritic. Every dog with a positive demodicosis should have fungal cultures done, because many of these puppies have more than one problem.

I have seen puppies with localized demodicosis, staph intermedius, and fungal infections concurrently. These must be treated with the appropriate drugs; however, one must keep in mind that all of these organisms are a normal inhabitant of the skin, albeit, at a much lower population.

A much more serious condition, generalized demodicosis, usually presents as multifocal to diffuse alopecia, with varying degrees of alopecia, grayish skin discoloration, erythema, scaling, and lichenification. These dogs are more prone to pruritis as there is usually a secondary superficial or deep pyoderma (infection) or a secondary fungal infection. Bacterial culture and sensitivity should always be performed on dogs that have weeping, draining lesions. I have routinely cultured both pseudomones and staph intermedius bacteria in such animals. These dogs frequently have to be put on life-saving antibiotics for a month or more.

There is no doubt that dogs with generalized demodicosis have severe cell-mediated immune dysfunction. Some researchers believe that there is an autosomal recessive mode of inheritance for this disease.[2] I have also seen this in dogs that have undergone immunosuppressive therapy for neoplastic or autoimmune diseases. Whether the symptoms are demodicosis, bacterial or fungal infections, or all of the above at the same time, these are all different symptoms of the same root cause of a derangement of the immune system.

There are many factors that will cause "derangement" of the immune system. Some of these may include vaccinosis, dead and devitalized food, chemicals in food, pesticides, herbicides, corticosteroids, stress, and genetics (purebred dogs).

These animals require a thorough work-up, a complete blood panel, and urinalysis; plus, their thyroid gland must be checked.

Treatments are frequently long-term and require patience by

both clinician and guardian. Western treatments include antibiotics, shampoos, and mitaban dips. Some dermatologists suggest using Ivermectin orally for up to three months.[3] Collies and other herding-type breeds should not be given Ivermectin. I personally have never used it because I believe the body does not need another xenobiotic to detoxify.

The most important part of the treatment is the immune modulation that must be implemented. During treatment, puppies must be taken off of all commercial foods and put on a live raw food diet that includes meat, vegetables, raw eggs, raw milk (if available), flax oil, fruit, raw bones, and whole grains. If palatability is a problem at first, then add broth or soup.

I also give all immune compromised patients weekly injections of Staphage Lysate (SPL)® to boost the TH_1 subset. I have used Staphylococcus Aureus Phage Lysate® in both dogs and cats for years and have never seen any side effects. It is made of staph aureus, a bacteriophage (virus that parasitizes bacteria), and saline. It was originally developed fifty years ago for humans with cancers. Physicians are no longer able to get SPL for their human patients; however, veterinarians are fortunate to have access to this valuable tool. It is routinely used for staph pyoderma in dogs as an adjunct to antibiotic therapy.[4] I have used staph lysate injections in such diseases as chronic allergies, asthma, bronchitis, infections, and cancers. Most patients respond within one month of weekly injections.

At Highlands Veterinary Hospital, I also routinely employ the use of biological response modifying herbs (see chapter 6) to treat skin diseases and acupuncture to expedite the healing process. Many dogs can be saved by employing a number of different modalities, and especially immune modulation. These dogs want to live, and we must be patient and give them a chance.

BACTERIAL AND FUNGAL DISEASES

Pyoderma is the term commonly used when defining the bacterial infections in dogs and cats. It is common in the canine and less so in the feline. An animal can certainly possess more than one pathological problem at one time. For example, pruritis (itching) can be caused by atopy (an allergy), external parasites, bacterial infections, fungal infections, and food allergies. I have seen pets that possessed four out of five abnormalities simultaneously.

Pyotraumatic dermatitis or "hot spots" can be caused by one or more of the aforementioned etiologies. Many cats exhibit "milliary dermatitis" and severe pruritis but no visible external parasites. I have diagnosed the majority of these cats with dermatophytosis or ringworm. Due to the self-mutilation, they have a secondary bacterial infection. However, it is extremely important to emphasize that the bacterial and fungal infections are not the primary etiology; they are secondary to a dysregulated or unbalanced and suppressed immune system.

These bacterial and/or fungal infections are normal inhabitants of the canine and feline skin and ears. However, when the situation presents itself, these organisms flourish with an increased population, and the vicious cycle ensues with pruritis.

The most common bacteria is staphylococcus intermedius, which inhabits both the canine and feline skin.[5] Pseudomonas are most commonly isolated from dogs with acute otitis extrerna or ear infection.

Budding yeast known as malassezia pachydermatis is a normal part of the skin flora; however, it is opportunistic and will lead to pathological signs when a primary disease alters the skin's microenvironment (temperature, humidity, and fats). With lowered immunological defenses, malassezia organisms can proliferate. The inflammatory mediators produced by proliferating yeast initiate the clinical signs observed. Remember, animals can possess multiple clinical signs from multiple etiologic factors.

Clinical signs of malassezia include generalized pruritis, alopecia, erythema, hyperpigmentation and lichenification, especially on dorsal, ventral, neck, axillary, inguinal, and perianal areas. The skin has a leather-like feel to the touch, but with correct treatment, the skin will revert back to soft, supple, and pink skin. Once again, these are normal inhabitants but at a much higher population.

Periodically young puppies will develop pustules at inguinal and abdominal areas and will be excessively pruritic. This is easily treated with antibiotics, antibacterial shampoos, and immune modulators. They will usually respond within two to three weeks.

Breeds such as the Sharpie or other short-haired breeds that are infected will have a "moth-eaten" appearance. This is called superficial folliculitis and is treated with antibiotics, shampoos, and immune modulators. These are long-term patients and must be put on a raw food diet as well. Processed foods must be eliminated. They should only be minimally fed with the bulk being raw meat, vegetables, raw milk, raw eggs, and raw bones.

Superficial fungal skin infections are extremely common in dogs and cats. There are three species of fungi that are mainly responsible for clinical signs. The three species of fungi (microsporum canis, microsporum gypseum, and trichophyton mentagrophytes) are responsible for most fungal skin infections (ringworm). Cats are more contagious to humans than are dogs. Ninety-five percent of the animals that I have cultured showed positive for fungal or yeast growth. Frequently the only clinical signs observed were variable degrees of itching. Many cats were misdiagnosed as having "milliary dermatitis," and dogs were misdiagnosed as having "allergies." Remember, many diseases can have overlapping clinical signs. Every dog and cat with pruritis can also possess a fungal infection. Any pet with a bacterial and/ or fungal infection has a compromised immune system. The initial treatments will include anti-infective drugs along with immune modulators and appropriate topicals (sprays, shampoos, and ointments).

Dermatophytes (fungi) normally inhabit the soil and can be found consistently on the hair and skin of outdoor pets. Infection is usually acquired from direct contact with contaminated soil, and once infected, an animal can transmit the fungus to other animals and humans.

Chronic pyodermas in the canine patient is common and should be viewed as a long-term problem. These patients are severely immune compromised and often will present with demodex and fungal infections. Treatment consists of acupuncture, raw food diet, Staphage Lysate injections, and various immune modulating herbs. In addition, appropriate anti-infective agents and topicals are important. Well-meaning people with "purist" intentions may argue that antibiotics will further compromise the immune system. However, one must realize that these infections frequently become systemic and life threatening.

All chronic pyoderma patients must have their thyroid gland evaluated; frequently, they are found to have a hypothyroid condition and must be placed on thyroid supplementation. There is more on hypothyroidism in chapter 10.

Let me emphasize that any life-threatening bacterial or fungal infection must be treated with the appropriate anti-infective agents along with an immune-enhancing protocol. I have seen many pets, which have been placed on anti-infective agents only, exhibit marginal or temporary success—and then relapse. Once diet change and immune-enhancing protocols were instituted, these animals were cured of their disease. Many animals that were destined to die or be euthanized were saved by, as I like to call it, the "Immune Package." The majority of diseases that I see at Highlands Veterinary Hospital are due to immune dysregulation. In an epidemic, the individuals with a strong "biological terrain," as researchers call it, will survive and the weaker will perish.

ALLERGIC AND IMMUNE-MEDIATED DISEASES

Allergy refers to a complex response to certain agents called allergens. Allergens produce a rapid physiological change that can result in asthma, sinus congestion, pruritis (itching hot spots), otitis externa (ear infections), paw licking and chewing, vomiting, and diarrhea. The unifying feature of allergy responses, which was identified in 1966, is involvement of the IgE system. IgE is one group of antibodies, which specifically attaches to cells located mostly in the skin and lining of the stomach, lungs, and upper respiratory airways. When the allergen binds to the antibodies, histamine and other chemicals are released from mast cells. This triggers the specific allergy symptoms through dilation of vessels, leakage of fluids from the vessels, and muscular tightening.

At the molecular level, the central factor is that leukocytes from patients with atopic dermatitis have decreased cyclic adenosine monophosphate (cAMP) levels due to increased cAMP-phosphodiesterase (enzyme that destroys cAMP) activity and a decreased level of beneficial prostaglandin precursors. The lack of intracellular cAMP results in increased histamine release and decreased bactericidal activity.[6] This starts a vicious cycle as the defective bactericidal activity could reflect an insufficient activation of the alternate complement pathway, an important part of the immune response. As we will later see, there are immune modulators that restore cAMP levels and thus the alternate complement pathway. The defects in immune function, coupled with intense scratching and the predominance of pathogenic staphylococcus in the skin flora of these patients, lead to the susceptibility to staph infections. There are also cell-mediated immunity defects that lead to increased susceptibility to cutaneous yeast and fungal infections. It is interesting that these patients' symptoms could have a cyclical effect; during clinical remission, cell-mediated immunity is normalized and becomes abnormal during recurrence of the dermatitis.[7]

It is important to realize that initially the immune system developed an allergy response to help the body deal with parasitic infections. As "survival of the fittest" goes, animals who could mount an effective response against parasite infections and survive had a greater chance of living a long life and bearing young. In areas of the world where parasite infection is common, the immune defense mechanism is effective at ensuring survival. In locations where parasites are not prevalent, the body reacts more readily to not-so-dangerous invaders (allergens).[8]

In many ways, the only difference between allergies and autoimmune disease is the target of the immune system's misdeeds.

Both create an imbalance in the immune system that makes it overreact. When the inflammatory response is directed against foods, pollens, or molds, it is called an allergic reaction. If it is directed against the joints, it may cause the autoimmune disease called rheumatoid arthritis. Similarly, if a zealous immune system goes after brain tissue, it may cause multiple sclerosis in humans, another autoimmune disease. In autoimmunity, the target is the body's own tissues, whereas with allergy, it is some foreign substance (pollen).

A balanced immune system normally distinguishes friend from foe and only attacks foreign invaders, avoiding the body's own tissues. A healthy immune system relies on B cells to produce antibodies that will destroy invading bacteria, viruses, fungi, and parasites before they get a chance to enter the healthy cells of the body. T cells are the immune cells that control and regulate the immune response or the call to battle. T cells are divided into two groups: helper T cells and cytotoxic T cells. The helper T cells are then broken down into two further groups called TH_1 helper cells and TH_2 helper cells. These cells have specific functions, and each type releases certain immune factors that help or hinder the immune response as required. When the TH_1 and TH_2 cells are in balance, health is maintained. If an overabundance of one or a deficiency of the other occurs, disease sets in. TH_1 helper cells release interleukin-2 and gamma interferon. TH_2 releases interleukin-4, interleukin-6, and interleukin-10, which enhance the ability of B cells to produce antibodies.[9]

If there is a reduction in the number or activity of TH_1 cells, natural killer cell activity, the first line of defense against invaders, is decreased. When TH_2 is elevated, an overabundance of antibodies is produced, which causes inflammation.

With a compromised immune system, many opportunistic invaders such as viruses, intracellular parasites, and bacteria have devised a mechanism of avoiding detection in the body by taking up residence inside healthy cells. B cells are often unable to mount an antibody assault once the invader is hiding in a host cell. The immune system has evolved to deal with most of these types of invaders by harnessing the power of cytotoxic T cells.

Cytotoxic T cells are told to become killing machines by TH_1 cells so that they can destroy any invader that has been able to get into a healthy cell. To get at the disease-causing organism hiding in the cell, cytotoxic T cells have to kill the host cell as well.

The immune system is finely tuned to adapt to changes that occur either when a virus or bacteria invades or when a cancer cell is lurking. When the TH_1 arm of the immune defense system is deficient, natural killer cell activity is reduced, infection and disease result, and chronic inflammation and eventually tissue damage (as seen in autoimmune disease) is inevitable.

Factors that lead to allergies and autoimmune diseases are complex and varied. They include:

1. Genetics

2. Dead and devitalized food (processed)

3. Over vaccinations (modified live viruses?)

4. Chemicals in the environment (xenobiotics)

5. Drugs (cortisone, immunosuppressive medications)

6. Stress

7. Viruses, bacteria, parasites, yeast, and fungi

It is apparent that both allergies and autoimmune diseases have the same root cause—an imbalance of the immune system. As you can see, the immune system is extremely complex, and one must rebalance the immune system to get a long-term cure and not just symptomatic relief or a quick fix with cortisone or other immunosupressive drugs such as azathioprine. If these drugs must be used, they should be used for short-term therapy only, while the body is getting symptomatic relief and being built up by immune-enhancing long-term therapies. I only use cortisone as a last resort, and 99 percent of the time I refrain from its usage.

Remember, by modulating the immune system and increasing TH_1 cells, which promote the secretion of interleukin-2 and gamma interferon, antibodies are down regulated along with severe inflammatory reactions.

All dogs should have a thorough blood work-up including thyroid function. It is well known that highly allergic dogs have a low thyroid function, which further compromises their condition.[10] All dogs and cats must have skin scrapings and fungal cultures taken because many will have concurrent dermatophytosis. Because staph infections are also pruritic, bacterial infections must be treated with appropriate antibiotics for a minimum of two to three weeks. Note that some cats show respiratory or asthmatic conditions and not skin diseases. These asthmatic patients also have severely compromised immune systems and must be built up.

I have not found allergy testing and desensitization to be cost effective. I believe these are a waste of time and money and often provide conflicting results. A more time-efficient and cost-effective immunotherapy would rebalance the TH_1 and TH_2 cells with a preferential bias toward TH_1 subset. In this way, we get inhibition of interleukin-3 (IL-3) and interleukin-4 (IL-4)-dependent IgE production. Secondly, the activity of mast cells is reduced because of a lack of IL-3 dependent activation, a reduced local production of IgE, and a decreased production of histamine-releasing factors.[11] The theory of the mechanisms of action of desensitization is unproven, and no benefits have been found in circulating IgG and IgE antibodies with treatment. When atopic individuals are tested, vets often will see an increase in the serum concentration of allergen-specific IgG. These IgG antibodies are thought to act as "blocking" antibodies by combining with circulating allergens to form immune complexes incapable of causing mast cell degranulation.[12] The measurement of IgG concentration has no predictive value and does not accurately correlate to clinical efficacy of desensitization therapy.

Another change seen with desensitization is an increase in both circulating and bound allergen-specific IgE. The initial rise in IgE is not harmful and, with long-term desensitization, will decrease but never be eliminated. In one study, it was found that IgE antibody concentration may not correlate with clinical improvement; and in any one patient, clinical efficacy may be achieved with a decrease, no change, or an increase in the concentration of IgE.[13] Desensitization is an inconsistent and a less than reliable technique to modulate the immune system. As I previously mentioned, the cell-mediated arm of the immune system is the crucial aspect of the immune system.

The most common clinical sign in dogs with atopy seen at Highlands Veterinary Hospital is chronic ear infections—inflamed, swollen and painful ears. With time, the ear canal becomes hyperplastic due to chronic inflammation, which inhibits air from getting down the canal. Microbes such as staph, pseudonomes, and yeast flourish and grow, which further inflames the ears. One or both ears can be infected. The ears will be quite painful and malodorous with varying degrees of dark, waxy debris or purulent discharge. Thorough cleaning and disinfection of the ears must be done on a regular basis along with the use of an antibacterial/antiyeast topical. Although bacteria and yeast are normal inhabitants of the ears, they can become overgrown due to the allergy and inflammation in infected pets. Long-term treatment must include biological response modifiers along with a raw food diet. Antibiotics may be used on a short-term basis; however, it is best to refrain from using corticosteroids. Long-term compromised immune systems may lead to a variety of serious diseases such as cancers. The best treatment is prevention; by enhancing the immune system, these pets will be healthier, happier, and much better off in the long run.

FOOD ALLERGIES

Lately, food allergies have become a "hot" topic in veterinary medicine. Food allergies can mimic other skin diseases; so a good thorough diagnostic work-up is imperative. The most common clinical sign of food allergy is generalized pruritis or itching.[14] Almost any body part can be affected including, and especially, the feet and ears. In cats, pruritis is more localized around the head area. Often they will have a secondary pyoderma or a pyotraumatic dermatitis (hot spot). Concurrent gastrointestinal signs may accompany dermatologic signs or GI signs such as colitis, bloody stool, fecal mucus, and flatus.

The best and only reliable diagnostic food allergy tool is a food elimination diet. Again, I must reiterate that the main problem is the ingestion of dead, devitalized, enzymeless food, which causes gastrointestinal leukocytosis. These pets must be fed a strict homemade raw food diet. If this is impractical, then incorporate raw food with the processed food as much as possible.

Blood tests for food allergies are expensive and unreliable. They should never be used as a criterion to eliminate food from the diet. A number of laboratories use an ELISA (enzyme immuno assay) panel to test for the presence of IgE or IgG. The premise behind this testing is that high circulating levels of antibodies are correlated with clinical food allergy signs and symptoms. The ELISA test itself involves coating well plates with food antigens, adding a patient's sera, and looking for an antigen/antibody interaction. This may be convenient for both clinician and patient; however, it is fraught with problems. These problems include reliability in testing, an arguable theory behind the testing, and the prevalence of treatments prescribed by these testing laboratories based solely on laboratory test results. A 1998 study by Bastyr University found many inconsistencies with food allergy testing involving three laboratories.[15] They found enormous problems in the preparation of the antigens (food). All foods are coated with microorganisms. Microorganisms have many antigens that are highly immunogenic. Most humans and animals have circulating immunoglobulins to a number of common microbes. As these microbes are in the wells, the serum may certainly react to these microbes or pesticides or even organic solvents used. Each well may possess many antigens and not just the food in question.

This certainly will give the possibility of false positive results.

An important point is that we may be depriving pets of good wholesome nutrition on the basis of unreliable test results. In my opinion, food allergy testing has no scientific basis and is not a holistic way to prescribe foods. Remember, the closer to the natural source food is, the healthier it will be; the more food is processed, the less healthy it will be. I once heard a saying, "The whiter the bread, the quicker you're dead." Processed food is for convenience and to keep one from starvation—not for good health.

NATURAL TREATMENTS FOR SKIN DISEASES

The main treatments for immune-mediated diseases are biological response modifiers (see chapter 6), raw food diets, and neutroceuticals with natural anti-inflammatory properties. The following are just a few herbs I have used with success.

Boswellia

Boswellia is but one of many beneficial herbs in an ancient therapeutic system known as Ayurveda. For more than 1,500 years, this valued herb has been used in India for its anti-inflammatory, anti-arthritic, and antipain properties.[16] Boswellic acids have shown to effectively shrink inflamed tissues, the underlying cause of pain in many conditions. These acids reduce inflammation and free radical activity by counteracting the effects of leukotrienes via the inhibition of 5-lipoxygenase pathway.

Curcumin

This is a common spice used in Indian cuisine with potent medicinal properties. Turmeric rhizome is used as a major ingredient in curry powder. It is used to preserve freshness of curry and various other foodstuffs. Turmeric spice has been reported to have potent antioxidant properties.[17] Tumeric contains an orange-yellow coloring matter with one of its constituents curcumin, though there are several curcuminoids, which have synergetic effects. Curcumin has been shown to have potent anti-inflammatory effects via inhibiting 5-lipoxygenase activity as well as the 12-lipoxygenase and cyclooxygenase activity.[18] Curcumin has also shown anticarcinogenic effects, and it is theorized that it is an antioxidant.

Feverfew

Feverfew has become a popular recommendation as a prophylactic treatment for migraine headaches in humans. Research studies have determined that parthenalides inhibit the production of prostaglandins, fatty acids that help control inflammation and body temperature. This inhibition of prostaglandins results in reduction in inflammation, decreased secretion of histamines, decreased activation of inflammatory cells, and a reduction of fever. Feverfew acts more like cortisone than aspirin or NSAIDs.[19] For feverfew to be effective, the parthenolide content must be standardized. I have used a feverfew product with a content of 600 mg per capsule to successfully treat a number of inflammatory and painful conditions in dogs and cats. When I get a headache, I ingest two capsules, and within fifteen minutes, my headache is gone. Due to its tonic effects on vascular smooth muscles, I have also used feverfew in cerebral vascular accidents (CVA) with success.

Flax Seeds

I have been using flax seeds and flax seed oil for a dozen years with remarkable results. Dogs accept flax oil readily, while cats seem to prefer crushed flax seeds or powder. I have used flax seeds for a number of inflammatory conditions ranging from allergies, colitis, autoimmune diseases, kidney disease, and cancers.

There are no magic bullets to good heath; however, essential fatty acids from a number of sources, especially flax seeds, play an important part. Other good sources are salmon (wild), sardines, trout, halibut, deer, elk, raw milk, and raw eggs.

Figure 7.1

Percentage of Omega-3 Fatty Acids in Fish and Meats

FOOD (PER 100 GRAMS OF MEAT)	OMEGA-3 FATTY ACIDS (%)
1. Salmon (wild)	4.65
2. Sardines (canned)	4.35
3. Trout	3.44
4. Halibut	2.84
5. Deer	2.89
6. Elk	2.76
7. Catfish	2.52
8. Lamb	1.81
9. Bison	1.63
10. Salmon (canned)	0.95
11. Chicken	0.93
12. Salmon (farmed)	0.87
13. Tuna (canned)	0.20

Flax is one of the most ancient of useful herbs. It is also one of the oldest continuously cultivated plants in history. Its Latin name, *Linum Usitatissimum*, means "most useful." From prehistoric times to the present, flax has been a source for food, fiber (linen), and oil. It has been used in herbal preparations. Fortunately, flax is quite nutritious and is used in cereal and bakery products. I regularly sprinkle flax seeds (powder) in cereal with raw milk to have a nutritious breakfast.

I commonly use flax seed oil in allergies and dry skin. How do essential fatty acids, which are found in flax oil, fit in the optimum health picture for both humans and pets alike? There exists an important relationship between the types and amount of fats in an animal's diet and its overall health and development. Essential nutrients are nutrients that cannot be manufactured by the body, so they must be supplied in the diet as food or supplements. There are two essential fatty acids: alpha-linolenic acid (omega-3) and linoleic acid (omega-6) fatty acid. If we get our omega-3 oils from wild fish or game, it comes in the form of EPA (eicosapantaenoic acid). Alpha-linolenic acid (omega-3) is present in small amounts in many oils, but highest in hemp and flax oils.

In the wild, herbivorous animals obtain the two essential fatty acids in plant foods that they eat. Essential fatty acids are primary components of cells and are readily incorporated in the tissues of these animals. Carnivorous animals, on the other hand, obtain these important nutrients by eating the essential fatty acid-rich tissues of their prey.

Though somewhat controversial, the ratio of omega-6 and omega-3 fatty acids supplied in the diet is equally important.[20] The ratio of essential fatty acids found in the diets of nondomestic animals equals 4 to 1 ratio of omega-6 to omega-3 fatty acids. Interestingly, these animals do not suffer from advanced degenerative diseases common in domestic animals.

Unfortunately, in today's society everyone wants fast convenient foods found in paper packaging and cans. This is a serious mistake, as the health of our companions pays the price due to poor nutrition. I bet a high percentage of a veterinarian's income is due to the devastating effect of feeding our pets dead and devitalized food. Modern manufacturing of pet and animal foods has caused an overabundance of omega-6 fatty acids, at the expense of the omega-3 fatty acids. Oils rich in omega-3 fatty acids (flax and hemp) are purposely avoided by animal food manufacturers because, unless protected from light, heat, and oxygen, they go rancid, lessening the shelf life and palatability of the food product. Therefore, our pets become deficient in these vital nutrients.

It is important to realize just how these nutrients play a role in health and disease. Most vegetable oils are high in omega-6 fatty acids. The omega-6 oils are converted into two different kinds of prostaglandins, hormone-like substances with powerful effects on our cells. The series-1 prostaglandins from omega-6 oils are anti-inflammatory and have a wide range of other health effects. Series-2 prostaglandins, on the other hand, are inflammatory and increase the tendency of our blood to clot. The body prefers to make series-1 prostaglandins out of dietary omega-6 oils, and with a healthy natural diet, only makes enough of the series-2 prostaglandins to maintain a healthy inflammatory response to infection and parasites. Drugs such as aspirin and corticosteroids act by suppressing the effects of these series-2 prostaglandins.

Humans and animals also require a third kind of prostaglandin, the series-3 prostaglandins from omega-3 oils, which are also anti-inflammatory and have other health benefits. If given the correct nutrients, the body has the ability to launch an inflammatory response, but has two substances—series-1 and series-3 prostaglandins—that will control and moderate that response so it does not get out of hand. Like the immune system, these three substances have to be in balance.

The metabolism of essential fatty acids is complex and is summarized in figure 7.2.

The question arises as to why I do not use fish oil products. A number of studies have raised the question of safety in the usage of fish oils.[21, 22] Fish oils tend to get rancid quickly and are contaminated with toxic derivatives known as peroxides. However, an acceptable stabilized fish oil produced by Eskimo-3 will stay fresh for at least nine months. Flax oil capsules are also to be avoided, because they too become rancid quickly.

Flax oil should be stored in the refrigerator in an opaque, tightly closed bottle with an expiration date printed on the bottle.

Ginger

Ginger is a versatile and safe herb. I have used it for a number of inflammatory ailments. Most of the traditional uses have involved the gastrointestinal tract. Most humans use it for nausea and vomiting. Ginger seems to stimulate digestion by keeping the intestinal muscles "toned."[23] Ginger also improves the production and secretion of bile from the liver and gallbladder. I have had great success using ginger to treat inflammatory bowl disease, as well as excess gas. Ginger also excels as an anti-inflammatory. A number

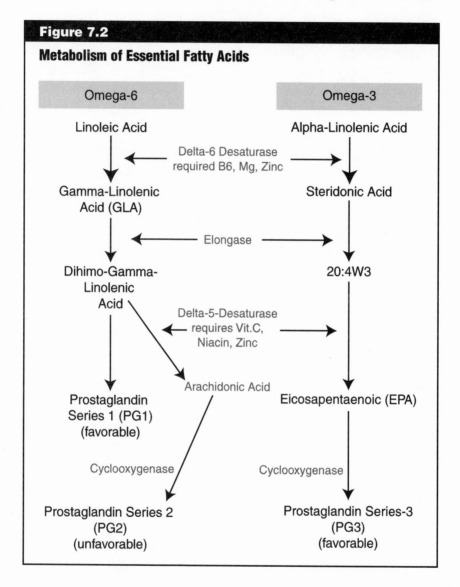

Figure 7.2

Metabolism of Essential Fatty Acids

Omega-6 | Omega-3

Linoleic Acid | Alpha-Linolenic Acid

Delta-6 Desaturase required B6, Mg, Zinc

Gamma-Linolenic Acid (GLA) | Steridonic Acid

Elongase

Dihimo-Gamma-Linolenic Acid | 20:4W3

Delta-5-Desaturase requires Vit.C, Niacin, Zinc

Arachidonic Acid

Prostaglandin Series 1 (PG1) (favorable) | Eicosapentaenoic (EPA)

Cyclooxygenase | Cyclooxygenase

Prostaglandin Series 2 (PG2) (unfavorable) | Prostaglandin Series-3 (PG3) (favorable)

of pruritic dogs have responded quite well to ginger.

In the Ayurvedic system of medicine, ginger is commonly used for inflammatory joint diseases. It has been shown that ginger counters the formation of pro-inflammatory substances such as leukotrienes and certain prostaglandins.[24]

I use a product that is standardized at 20 percent for gingerols and shogaols. If a product is not standardized, it is probably of inferior quality and will not work as well.

Licorice

Corticosteroids are considered by many to be among the great wonder drugs of the twentieth century. Encompassing a family of similar chemicals including hydrocortisone, prednisone, predniso-lone, triamcinolone, and depo-medral, these drugs all mimic the effects of natural hormones produced by the adrenal glands.

These powerful drugs have many actions, but the overall effect is to decrease inflammation. Taken by pill or injection, they can suppress the symptoms of asthma, arthritis, pruritis, and many other inflammatory diseases. The important word is "suppress" and not "cure." Cure can only be achieved by a totally holistic approach.

Licorice has been used in a multitude of Chinese formulas without any side effects. However, when used as a single herb, caution must be used. As it turns out, many of the beneficial effects of licorice root result from its ability to increase blood levels of corticosteroids. It does this by blocking the enzyme 5-beta-reductase, which is responsible for breaking down these hormones prior to their elimination. That same enzyme also breaks down a hormone called aldosterone, which acts to raise blood pressure and increase potassium loss through the urine. Thus, by raising aldosterone levels in the body, licorice indirectly increases blood pressure.[25]

I only use licorice in Addison's disease, or when reducing the dosages of corticosteroids in patients that have been taking these drugs for extended periods. It is important to "wean" patients off of corticosteroids slowly over a period of weeks and not to go "cold turkey" or the patient may go into shock due to severe adrenal suppression.

If one must use synthetic corticosteroids for short periods of time, licorice may be of benefit in allowing corticosteroids to be used at a much lower dosage. This is true complementary medicine where a patient may reap the rewards of both worlds.

I have developed a magnolia flower formula consisting of ginkgo, licorice, perilla, scute, tuessilago, siler, angelica, akebia, asarum, ma-huang, morus, cimicifuga, and cnidium. This formula has helped both dogs and cats with chronic sinusitis, bronchitis, nasal congestion, asthma, and chronic obstructive pulmonary disease.

Quercetin

Quercetin is widely distributed in the plant kingdom and is the most abundant of all the flavonoids, which are found in the rinds and skins of fruits and vegetables. It also happens to be the most pharmacologically active of all the flavonoids. Flavonoids, as a rule, are antioxidants, and a number of quercitin's effects appear to be due to its antioxidant activity.

I have used a combination of flavonoids for their anti-inflammatory activity. Unfortunately, when used as isolated nutrients, they must be used with enzymes to enhance absorption. Quercetin inhibits the inflammation-producing enzyme (cyclooxygenase) and its subsequent inflammatory mediators (leukotriens and prostaglandins).[26,27] Quercetin also stabilizes mast cells and basophils.[28]

Quercetin in clinical practice does possess some anti-inflammatory and anti-histaminic effects; however, its effects may not be realized for several weeks. Though dogs and cats produce vitamin C, under times of disease and stress, it is important to provide it in the diet. I am not referring to ascorbic acid, which has no healing ability, but to fruits and vegetables. Real vitamin C from foods has bioflavonoids as part of its make-up. When using these nutrients in an isolated manner, they seem to act more as drugs than nutrients.

I have used quercetin in atopy, autoimmune diseases, inflammatory bowel disease, and asthma. Interestingly, guercitin has been shown to have anticarcinogenic effects.[29] Quercetin is abundant in the brassica family of vegetables as well as herbs such as ginkgo and elderberry. This may explain in part ginkgo's therapeutic

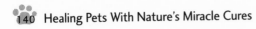

effects. Many bioflavonoids have also shown to have antiviral effects as well.

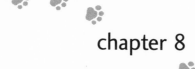

chapter 8

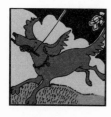

Arthritis and How to Keep Your Pet Moving

THE MOST COMMON FORM OF ARTHRITIS IN PETS IS OSTEOARTHRITIS, which is also called degenerative joint disease. Osteoarthritis is mainly seen in elderly large breed dogs, though I've also treated it in dogs as young as one year old, in golden retrievers and German shepherds. There are certainly genetic factors involved, and prospective owners should consult with breeders as to the status of the parents.

Response to pain varies with individual dogs. Some dogs will exhibit severe pain with mild arthritis, while others will exhibit mild pain symptoms with severe arthritis.

Weight-bearing joints such as the hips, elbows, and knees are most often affected by degenerative changes associated with osteoarthritis. Specifically, extensive cartilage destruction is followed by cartilage hardening and the formation of large spurs in the joint margins. Cartilage serves an important role in joint function. Its gel-like nature provides protection to the ends of joints by acting as a shock absorber. Degeneration of the cartilage is the hallmark of osteoarthritis. With this degeneration comes inflammation, pain, deformity, and diminished range of motion in the joint.[1]

Arthritis of the knees is usually secondary to a cranial cruciate rupture. This can be prevented by new effective surgical techniques usually performed by surgical specialists.

Dogs suffering from hip dysplasia are often reluctant to jump or rise from their rear legs, have difficulty moving well, and may be hesitant to climb and descend stairs. These dogs may also be visibly distressed when their hips are touched or manipulated. They may have difficulty getting up after a long rest or favor one or both hind legs after extensive exercise. The muscle mass in the rear legs may be atrophied as well.

With arthritis of the elbows, the dog may "bop" the head up and down as it walks. In fact, I have encountered arthritic elbows so frequently that I suggest every older dog that is screened for hip dysplasia should also be screened for arthritic elbows.

Inflammation is the body's response to injury, infection, allergy, or degeneration. This response causes the tissue to swell and become irritated or even painful. Two types of inflammation can be experienced: acute and chronic. Acute inflammation occurs with an injury and results in pain that typically lasts only a short time. Chronic inflammation, on the other hand, can lead to constant debilitating pain and swelling, sometimes lasting for years.

When joints are strained or overworked, tiny cells around the joints release histamine and other bioactive compounds. These compounds cause the nearby capillaries to become permeable and expand (vasodilatation). Histamine warns the body that the injury has taken place. Next, phagocytes move to the affected area, bringing with them natural inflammatory chemicals that surround the joint, causing swelling and pain.

When inflammation occurs, the body's natural defense mechanisms respond by sealing off the injured site with a mesh-like fibrin barrier (small thread-like molecules). The fibrin barrier temporarily blocks nutrients from entering the area while the body tries to heal the injured site. Fibrin formation also leads to excess fluid retention at the injured site, causing pain, irritation, and swelling. With acute inflammation, in the case of injury or strain, the symptoms will most likely disappear in a short time (days to weeks). However, poorly healed inflamed tissue or reinjury of the joint may eventually lead to a chronic disability such as arthritis.

Certain pro-inflammatory chemicals not only cause chronic inflammation, but they can also encourage the weakening of collagen, the building block of connective tissue essential to the health of joints (including cartilage, ligaments, and tendons). When collagen breaks down, cartilage can no longer absorb shocks and ligaments lose their flexibility. In addition, an enzyme called hyaluronidase is released, which breaks down hyaluronic acid. Hyaluronic acid lubricates and cushions joints, and its degradation increases the irritation of joint components. This series of events causes movement to become stiff and painful, a condition recognized as arthritis.

Most of my patients have responded to a combination of acupuncture and herbs, though a small percentage were placed on low doses of nonsteroidal anti-inflammatories, also known as NSAIDs, in combination with herbs. Long-term high doses of NSAIDs have the potential to cause pathology of the liver and kidneys, and, of course, ulcers. So it is always advisable to use them as a last resort.

Besides the neutraceuticals (functional foods) I am about to discuss, I have also used the herbs in chapter 7 for their anti-inflammatory effects.

NATURAL REMEDIES FOR ARTHRITIS IN PETS

Arthred

Arthred, which is hydrolyzed collagen, is made up of a series of eighteen amino acids that are joined together in chains of peptide bonds. These amino acids are the same as those that make up the framework of cartilage cells, contributing to configuration, flexibility, and strength. Animals fed the active ingredients in arthred experience such significant cartilage growth, researchers could measure it with a ruler. In a controlled study done in 1993 at the clinical department of the Veterinary University in Hanover, Germany, significant increase in cartilage thickness was observed.[2] In one study 356 people suffering from arthritis in one or more joints (knees, hips, spine, or digits) took one tablespoon of arthred daily. Test results were based on subjective statements with 99.2 percent reporting "good" or "very good" results.[3] There were no side effects. Researchers concluded that arthred had the strongest pain-relieving effects in those suffering with arthrosis of the knees and finger joints. In another study, sixty patients with arthritis of the knees were treated with arthred for three months. At the end of the study, 75 percent of the patients were free of pain and 86 percent reported greater ease in climbing stairs.[4] In one double-blind study, fifty-two patients suffering from arthritis for at least five years took arthred or placebo for sixty days. For every type of pain studied, arthred was significantly more effective than the placebo.[5]

Practical clinical experience at Highlands Veterinary Hospital in hundreds of arthritic dogs shows arthred to alleviate pain and give greater mobility. As a side benefit, animals grew more luxurious coats, and there was expedited healing of skin diseases. In a vast majority of pets on arthred, we were able to either eliminate or drastically reduce both NSAIDs or steroids, thus reducing the possibility of side effects. Arthred is an odorless and tasteless powder, thus making it easily acceptable by both dogs and cats.

It is important to remember that when addressing joint problems, we are dealing with specialized cells called connective tissues. These are made up of several different structures: Collagen accounts for 50 percent of connective tissue. Proteoglycans, also called glycosaminoglycans, make up 30 percent of connective tissues. The remaining 20 percent of connective tissue mass is made up of chondrocytes, actually living cells that manufacture collagen.

In healthy cartilage tissue, an equilibrium exists between the collagen and the proteoglycans. They decompose and recreate at a certain rate. If this balance is upset, more cartilage is lost than created, and arthritis develops. Arthred helps to replenish cartilage cells.

Drynaria 12
Drynaria 12 is composed of drynaria, dipsacus, rehmannia, astragalus, millettia, tang-kuei, achyrenthes, eucommia, deer antler, cnidium, pine node, and asarum. This formula diminishes pain by increasing circulation to the joints. It also has analgesic and anti-inflammatory effects.

I have used this formula for years with tremendous results. Normally, I use Drynaria 12 with a chondroprotective (cartilage protector) neutraceutical.

Glucosamine Sulfate
Glucosamine sulfate is the building block from which the major Glycosaminoglycans (GAGs) are formed (chondroitin sulfate, dermatan sulfate, and hyoluronate). GAGs help keep joints functioning as well as repair damaged cartilage. Glucosamine sulfate is so important that it is found in virtually all body tissues including bones, tendons, ligaments, cartilage, synovial fluid, heart valves, blood vessel linings, and mucous membranes of the digestive, respiratory, and urinary tracts. It is a natural part of the "glue" that holds the body cells together. In short, the manufacture of glucosamine determines the amount of GAGs synthesized. The main physiologic function of glucosamine on joints is to stimulate the manufacture of substances necessary for proper joint function, such as GAGs. It is also responsible for stimulating joint repair.

Sulfur (see chapter 4) is an essential nutrient for joint tissue; it functions as a link with other molecules in a criss-cross fashion. It is this stabilized structure that helps give connective tissue its form, strength, resiliency, and shock-absorbing qualities. In addition to sulfur playing a critical role in the manufacture of GAGs, it has been shown that sulfur inhibits the various enzymes that lead to cartilage destruction in osteoarthritis (collagenase, elastase, and hyaluronidase).[6] Thus sulfur is a critical element; lack of sulfur will produce less GAG synthesis. Most of the efficacious research shows that glucosamine sulfate in its stabilized form is efficacious in osteoarthritis; however, other forms lack the extensive studies to support their use.[7] Glucosamine sulfate by itself does not act as a pain reliever or anti-inflammatory; rather it acts by initiating repair of damaged joint tissue.

I have been using stabilized glucosamine sulfate for a number of years with great success. Many products are not stabilized and thus lose their potency over time.

Liquidambar 15

Liquidambar 15 is composed of liquidambar, pyrola, geranium, cibotium, pterospermum, photinia, kadsura, morus twig, loranthus, chuan shan, rehmannia, myrrh, carthamus, persica, and achyranthes. This formula diminishes pain by combining the use of some herbs that increase circulation with others that have anti-inflammatory and analgesic effects. I use this formula with chondroprotective agents.

Lyprinol

Lyprinol is an oil extract made from perna canaliculus, also known as New Zealand green-lipped mussel. To the best of my knowledge, it appears that the active therapeutic agent in green-lipped mussel extract is eicosatetraenoic acid (ETA), a member of the omega-3 family of essential fatty acids (EFAs), found primarily in fish. Although this is a relatively new extract, it seems to have more potent biological activity than either eicosopentaenoic acid (EPA) or docosahexaenoic acid (DHA).

How does lyprinol (ETA) work in reducing inflammation? Biochemically speaking, an overabundance of arachidonic acid (omega-6) in the cells is one factor that can lead to painful inflammation, and inappropriate dietary intake of fats can produce this excess. This buildup of arachidonic acid can cause inflammation in two ways: by forming either too many leukotrienes (which initiate inflammation) or too many prostaglandins (hormones involved in the process of inflammation). Thus pain and inflammation ensue. Standard anti-inflammatory drugs work by inhibiting the formation of prostaglandins, but the fats in liprinol block the formation of leukotrienes. The advantage here is that the mussel extract can block or reduce inflammation without the serious side effects (intestinal bleeding, kidney failure) of conventional arthritic drugs.

Researchers in Australia at the University of Queensland tested liprinol's performance against other oils such as flax, evening primrose, and Norwegian salmon oils. In terms of blocking inflammation, lyprinol was 240 times more effective than Norwegian salmon oil, 300 times more potent than evening primrose oil, and 400 times more potent than flax oil.[8] What I found quite interesting, however, were the results when researchers compared liprinol (the extract) to green-lipped mussel in powdered form at 300 mg/kg. Inflammation was reduced by 97 percent, and when given liprinol at 5 mg/kg, inflammation was reduced by 91 percent. This demonstrates that liprinol was more potent than the powdered form of green-lipped mussel.

I found that liprinol takes about four weeks to "kick in"; however, it is safe and works quite well in a variety of inflammatory diseases. I use liprinol with chondroprotective agents for arthritis.

Perna Canaliculus (New Zealand Green-Lipped Mussel)

I have been using perna canaliculus as a chondroprotective agent for more than ten years with great results. It has been quite reliable, and hence, I am still administering it to dogs and cats alike. It is a whole food supplement, which contains complex proteins, natural vitamins, minerals, and enzymes that all work together to help repair and maintain connective tissue and joint function. Glycosaminoglycans (chondroitin-4-sulfate, dermatan sulfate, chondroitin-6-sulfate, heparin sulfate, chondroitin polysulfate, heparin, and hyaluronic acid) make up 10-15 percent of perna.

Perna seems to enhance the regenerative pathways of the cell, including the chondrocytes (cartilage cells) in the synovial membranes. It increases the biological uptake and production of natural substances such as the sulfated GAGs and hyaluronic acid, which are already present in healthy joints. Hyaluronic acid's key role is to help maintain proper lubrication and viscosity within the synovial cavity. GAGs stimulate the secretion of joint fluid, which increases the viscosity and reduces the level of damaging proteins in the joint. They also act to repair damaged cartilage by encouraging growth of collagen matrix.

Sea Cucumber

The reason sea cucumber is valuable is because it serves as a rich source of polysaccharide chondroitin sulfate (similar to perna), a well-known chondroprotective agent. I use this as I do perna canaliculus with equal benefit to both dogs and cats. Preliminary studies also suggest that it may possess antiviral and anticancer properties.[9]

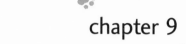

chapter 9

Digestive Tract Diseases and Processed Pet Food

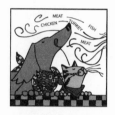

I BELIEVE THAT, IN ALL BUT A FEW CASES, THE MAJORITY OF GASTROINTES-
TINAL TRACT (GIT) PROBLEMS in dogs and cats are caused by the
ingestion of dead, enzymeless, and contaminated food. The dysfunction, discomfort, and disease associated with the GIT are the
result of local immune responses to processed foods. In nature,
food is meant to be digested by enzymes inherent within the food
itself; since modern society's processed food has no enzymes, the
pancreas must do most of the digestive work—a burden it was
never designed to carry alone. Processed food, as opposed to raw
enzyme-rich natural foods, will produce "digestive leukocytosis"
within the GIT. Pets that eat processed foods must be supplemented with enzymes to assist in digestion and allow more nutrients to be absorbed. Of course, there are other causes of digestive
tract diseases, ranging from viruses and bacteria to foreign objects. In this chapter, we look at what the digestive track does,
how it responds to attack, who the likely culprits are, and how
natural cures can help.

HOW THE GASTROINTESTINAL TRACT WORKS

The gastrointestinal tract is a long muscular tube that functions as the food processor for the body. The digestive system includes the following organs: the mouth and salivary glands, stomach, small and large intestines, liver, pancreas, and gallbladder. Irritation or inflammation of the various sections of the GIT is identified as gastritis (stomach), ileitis (small intestine), colitis (colon), hepatitis (liver), cholecystitis (gallbladder), and pancreatitis (pancreas).

The GIT is not a passive system; rather it has the capability to sense and react to the materials that are passed through it. Dogs and cats are carnivores and thus require a meat-based diet, as opposed to the grain-based diets so conveniently available on our grocery shelves.

The GIT breaks down food by first using mechanical means, such as chewing, and then by applying a host of complex chemical processes. These chemical processes include everything from saliva to colon microbes. Since the GIT is the point of entry for the body, everything eaten has an impact on the body. The food eaten and passed through the GIT contains nutrients as well as toxins. Toxins can be anything from preservatives, food additives, pesticides, and herbicides to specific foods that induce a reactive response by the GIT.

The process of digestion is accomplished with digestive chemicals, which are secreted from accessory glands located along the surface of the GIT. The two glands providing the majority of digestive chemicals utilized by the GIT are the liver and pancreas. The function of the liver is to control the food supply for the rest of the body by further processing the food molecules absorbed through the intestines. This is done by dispensing these food molecules in a controlled manner, and by filtering out toxins that may have passed through the GIT wall.

Another important function of the GIT is as a sensory organ. By rejecting foods through objectionable taste, vomiting, diarrhea, or any combination of these symptoms, the sensing capacity of the GIT can protect the body. The surface of the GIT, or mucosa, is part of a complex sensing system called the MALT (mucosa associated lymphatic tissue). MALT's immune sensors trigger responses such as nausea, vomiting, pain, and swelling. Vomiting and diarrhea are abrupt defensive responses to MALT sensing foods with a strong allergic or toxic component. This kind of food intolerance is responsible for many digestive problems. The GIT is connected to the brain via hormonal and neurotransmitter chemical communication.

The GIT is a muscular tube that contracts in a controlled rhythm to move food through the different sections (peristalsis). Strength and timing variations in the contractions can cause abdominal pain (cramping) and diarrhea (frequent contractions). When the contractions are slow and irregular, constipation may occur.

STOMATITIS

This is acute or chronic inflammation of the oral cavity. It is rarely seen in dogs but common in cats. When dogs have stomatitis, it is usually associated with bacterial infections; stomatitis in cats is associated with immune-mediated or viral infections.

In felines, systemic causes of oral lesions include metabolic diseases (kidney failure); infectious diseases, such as herpes, calicivinus, feline leukemia virus (FELV), and feline immunodeficiency virus (FIV); toxins; autoimmune diseases; and nutritional deficiencies. Tumors of the oral cavity must always be ruled out when suspected.

Clinical signs of oral inflammatory diseases include anorexia, dysphasia (difficulty swallowing), ptyalism (salivation), halitosis (bad breath), pain on opening the mouth, and pawing at mouth or face.

Lymphacytic-plasmacytic gingivitis and stomatitis are probably the most commonly seen feline oral soft-tissue diseases. Frequently biopsies are needed to differentiate these from squamous cell carcinoma, the most common feline oral tumor.[1]

These feline patients possess severe derangements of the immune system. Treatments must be directed at rebalancing the immune system with a natural raw food diet, biological response modifiers, neutraceuticals, and herbs with anti-inflammatory activity. Both veterinarian and guardian must have patience in dealing with this lifelong disease. With time, control and cure are possible. The immune system must be rebalanced to affect a cure. (See chapter 6 on the immune system and biological response modifiers and chapter 2 on nutrition.)

Long-term usage of glucocorticoids is discouraged. They provide only short-term symptomatic relief, not a cure. If corticosteroids are used, they should only be used along with biological response modifiers and in short-term low dosages to stimulate appetite and alleviate pain.

Eosinophylic granuloma complex is an ulcerative lesion usually seen on the upper lip of cats. Pure-breed cats, which may have limited genetic variability, are prone to autoimmune diseases. The more severe the autoimmune disease, the more unbalanced the immune system. There are no magic bullets for the treatment of these diseases. Only synergistic actions using a variety of modalities can affect a cure.

GASTRITIS (VOMITING)

Both acute and chronic gastritis is common in dogs and cats, and there are many potential causes. Frequently, in acute gastritis, the exact cause is never identified; however, the pet's history will lead one to a suspicious cause. The most common cause of acute gastritis is related to dietary indiscretion (ingestion of plants or garbage). The ingestion of foreign materials, plants and plant toxins, and hair causes gastritis by irritating the lining of the stomach. When in doubt, radiographs must be taken to rule out foreign objects. Such objects must be surgically or endoscopically removed. I have removed many foreign objects such as bones, tennis balls, and rocks that would have surely killed the pet if not removed surgically. Incidentally, most raw bones are safe and are easily digestible by both dogs and cats.

Many drugs have the potential to cause gastritis as well: non-steroidal anti-inflammatories, dexamethasone (steroid), and some antibiotics, to name a few. Certain infectious agents such as coronavirus, parvovirus, and canine distemper virus cause acute gastritis as well as diarrhea. Bacterial and parasitic infections may also cause acute gastritis. In fact, I have observed dogs that appeared to vomit on an empty stomach. When the dog was fed several small meals daily and just before bedtime, vomiting ceased. This is caused by reflux of duodenal fluid into the stomach (alkaline reflux gastritis), which may cause recurrent vomiting episodes of bile-stained fluid. I call this condition "sour stomach syndrome." Lastly, allergic reactions to a food antigen or impurities in the food may cause gastritis.

In chronic conditions, a thorough diagnostic work-up (blood panel, radiographs, ultrasound, endoscopy, barium study, and exploratory surgery) must be done to exclude neoplastic, metabolic, or autoimmune diseases.

Treatment is dependent upon identification of the cause. In many cases, simply putting the pet on a predominantly natural raw food diet cures the problem. Many pets will respond to a variety of herbs such as ginger, bioflavonoids, flax seeds, lyprinol, enzymes, and other neutraceuticals with anti-inflammatory effects. Drugs such as cimetidine (H_2 antagonist) must be used with caution because they often inhibit protein digestion and stimulate bacterial overgrowth. With a suspected bacterial infection or overgrowth of gastrointestinal microbes, antibiotics such as metronidazole are effective. Metronidazole is safe and effective, even if taken for several weeks; however, some rare neurological reactions have occurred at high doses. Neurological signs subside with removal of the drug. Many pets with chronic gastritis respond to biological response modifiers due to their compromised immune systems.

If food allergy is suspected, then an elimination diet must be performed using one protein source for four to six weeks.

GASTRIC DILATATION-VOLVULUS

Gastric dilatation-volvulus (GDV) occurs most commonly in giant breed, deep-chested dogs. The exact cause is unknown, but overeating, genetic factors, exercising immediately after eating, excessive drinking after or before exercise, and laxity of the gastrohepatic ligament make the list of potential culprits.

This is an acute life-threatening condition and must be dealt with surgically at once. Vomiting or attempting to vomit without the production of vomitus are common signs. The abdomen will appear enlarged and bloated. Remember, this is an emergency situation, and time is of the essence.

When surgically correcting this condition, I prefer to inject dimethylsulfoxide (DMSO) intravenously along with other treatments for shock prior to surgery. DMSO has greatly increased post-surgical survival of my patients. Its potent antioxidant, anti-inflammatory, and reperfusion attributes increase oxygen to vital organs.

Prevention is achieved by feeding small amounts of easily digestible foods several times daily. Large breed dogs should never be fed large meals at any one sitting.

HAIRBALLS

Though cats vomit frequently, one should not automatically assume that hairballs are the problem. Chronic vomiting in the feline patient must be thoroughly worked up diagnostically to rule out metabolic, neoplastic, autoimmune, and food intolerance conditions. Over-the-counter hairball medicines work quite well. I prefer a regimen of enzyme supplementation and crushed flax seeds added to food as viable alternatives. Offering good tasting and nutritious wheat grass is still another alternative for the elimination of hairballs in cats.

DYSBIOSIS

One of the best kept secrets in human and veterinary medicine is that the gastrointestinal tract is the largest immune organ in the body. When you think about this, however, it should not really come as much of a surprise. The intestinal lining has a huge surface area that separates the outer external world from the internal body. Nature has placed the body's defense system at a strategic location where potentially dangerous invaders or chemicals may enter the body. It does not require one to be a rocket scientist to realize that if this large, strategically placed immune system is not working up to par, then the ensuing lowered defenses may not be sufficient to keep the ecology of the intestinal tract in balance.

Our immune system can malfunction in at least three ways. First, it can be weakened so that it cannot mount an adequate response to invasion. In this immunosuppressed state, the body cannot fight off the usual stresses that accompany physical and psychological stress, cancer, and viral infections. Second, it can overreact or become hyper-responsive to normal stimuli, which is what occurs in asthma or atopy. Such hyperactivity not only uses up the immune reserves of the body, but it may cause immune reactions that create tissue injury. Third, it can set the stage for autoimmune reactions, wherein antibodies are made against our own tissues; this occurs in rheumatoid arthritis or lupus.

Regardless of the mechanism of immune malfunction, the end result is the same: abnormal host defense mechanisms that can lead to the development of dysbiosis. Dysbiosis is defined as a disordered microbial ecology that causes disease. This state may exist in the oral cavity, small intestine, or colon. In dysbiosis, organisms that do not normally cause infection, including bacteria, yeast, and protozoa, induce disease by producing toxins or altering the nutrition or immune responses of their host. Some of the toxic chemicals they produce are carcinogens, while others provoke an allergic response.[2]

Unfortunately, many of the microbial metabolic by-products and toxins can pass easily from the intestines into the blood. It is also wise to keep in mind that dysbiosis is not a disease *per se*. As a matter of fact, dysbiosis is usually found secondary to other diseases. Nevertheless, the presence of dysbiosis is clearly an abnormal situation and should not be overlooked when treating small or large intestinal diseases. Unlike the situation in man, both dogs and cats normally have a large number of small intestinal microbes. It is generally agreed that most of the microbes are of the anaerobic type. These organisms can be cultured, put into capsule form, and ingested into the intestinal tract, where they can reestablish a healthy ecological balance. These bacteria are termed "probiotics," because they support the microflora, in contrast to antibiotics, which kill the microflora. Many companies add a "prebiotic" to their probiotic mixture of microbes. Prebiotics consist of fibers, which nutritionally support the probiotic microbes.

Small intestinal bacterial overgrowth is common in dogs and cats and is usually seen secondary to dietary indiscretion, motility disorders, malfunctioning immunological defenses, or environmental toxins. Management must be directed at underlying causes as well as decreasing bacterial overgrowth with antibiotics such as metronidazole. Ingestion of plain yogurt or raw milk is helpful in the treatment of dysbiosis. Fructo-oligosaccharides (FOS) are short chain carbohydrates found in various plants. When consumed, they interfere with the ability of pathogenic bacteria to attach to the intestinal epithelium. Garlic, nutritional yeast, and artichoke are high in fructo-oligosaccharides.

INFLAMMATORY BOWEL DISEASE AND COLITIS

Chronic diarrhea generally involves two abnormal processes: One is insufficient absorption of water (and possibly fats and complex carbohydrates) from the intestines. The other is excessive intestinal peristalsis, which moves the fecal material through the intestines more rapidly than usual, reducing time for absorption of fluids and nutrients and passing the material to the rectum in a relatively short time.

For ease of simplicity, we will define inflammatory bowel disease (IBD) as a group of enteric diseases characterized by the infiltration of the small intestine, colon, or both by various cells of the immune system.

Pets with IBD usually have a history of chronic vomiting, diarrhea, or weight loss. Animals may or may not be anorectic, dehydrated, or have poor flesh. Diarrhea is often watery, but stools may be soft or semi-formed. Fresh blood or mucus may be present in individuals with colonic involvement. Melena (black stool) occurs in cases with either small intestine or gastric involvement. Vomiting is a common clinical sign, and most often occurs with no relationship to feeding.

Diagnostic work-up includes multiple fecal checks for parasites and giardia, trypsin-like immunoreactivity (TLI) for pancreatic enzyme activity, radiographs, barium study, endoscopy, complete blood profile, and exploratory surgery if needed to rule out cancer.

This is a disease of a fast-food society that places more importance on convenience than quality of food. IBD is poorly understood in allopathic medicine. It does not appear in wild dogs and cats, which eat raw unprocessed food, free of chemicals, pesticides, herbicides, preservatives, binders, and fillers. Evolution has not adapted the descendants of wolves or wild cats for fast, enzymeless, dead food. In fact, the raw meat eaten in the wild is "contaminated" by soil organisms. Soil-based organisms (SBOs) are a type of probiotic, which is a transient bacterial inhabitant of the gastrointestinal tract. A probiotic is a beneficial microorganism that limits the proliferation of disease-causing microbes by competitive exclusion in the gastrointestinal tract of humans and animals.[3] Among other functions, SBOs produce and release enzymes that sterilize the soil of putrefactive organisms, and thereby help prepare the soil to support new plant growth. Interestingly, it is these microbes that preserve the flesh of prey animals that are stored in the ground for later dining by predators. Additionally, SBOs have been shown to stimulate the body's production of alpha-interferon, B- and T-lymphocytes, and superoxide dismutase as well as to increase nutrient absorption.[4]

Over the years, researchers have sought to identify inflammatory bowel disease as an infectious process (bacterial, viral, parasitic, fungal, yeast). The problem may be that the infectious agent may be a component of the normal intestinal flora, which suddenly produces immunostimulatory toxins or becomes invasive as a direct result of sublethal doses of antibiotics. Antibiotics must be given for a minimum of five days at an appropriately high dose to kill the bacteria and to minimize the growth of resistant strains.

An overwhelming amount of evidence points to immune system disturbance in inflammatory bowel disease. However, I believe these disturbances are secondary to other factors such as food allergies, devitalized food, binders, fillers, preservatives, and other impurities in food. Though some gastroenterologists maintain this is an autoimmune disease, it is wise to remember that all autoimmune diseases have a root cause, and to affect a cure, one must look first to the diet. Treatment with immunosuppressive drugs will produce short-term symptomatic relief but not a long-term cure. However, one allopathic drug that I have used along with natural therapeutics is metronidazole. Its beneficial properties include broad-spectrum activity against anaerobic bacteria, antiprotozoal activity,[5] and potent inhibition of cell-mediated immunity.[6] Though side effects are rare, metronidazole has been associated with peripheral neuropathy in dogs. I have only seen one such case in a puppy, which was quickly resolved with the removal of the drug.

Natural treatments are the mainstay and most important treatments for inflammatory bowel disease. A natural raw food diet and biological response modifiers are the most important aspects of treatment for IBD. In addition, the following natural therapies help to cure these maladies.

Enzymes
Even a raw food natural diet will benefit from supplementation of digestive enzymes.

Probiotics

The reintroduction of desirable microflora also called "friendly bacteria" will help balance microflora in the body.

Glutamine

The amino acid glutamine is the principal fuel for the small intestine enterocytes. It is the most abundant amino acid in the bloodstream and is considered to be a "conditionally essential" amino acid.[7] Glutamine is a tri-peptide (glutamic acid, glycine, and cysteine). This potent intracellular antioxidant has glutathione-enhancing effects, which are necessary for liver detoxification.[8] Glutamine also serves as a precursor molecule for glucosamine synthesis, which is essential for mucin synthesis (the protective mucus layer in the gut).

Fiber

I prefer to use crushed flax seeds. Flax seeds are also high in omega-3 fatty acids, which have natural and safe anti-inflammatory effects. Soluble fiber decreases the pH of the intestines, encourages the growth of beneficial organisms, and suppresses growth of pathogenic organisms such as clostridium difficile.[9]

Lyprinol

Lyprinol is an extract from New Zealand green-lipped mussels (perna canaliculus). It contains a unique group of fatty acids, estimated to be about two hundred times as potent as cold-water fish oil, for anti-inflammatory effects.

Bioflavonoids

Quercetin and other bioflavonoids have been shown to stabilize mast cells. Mast cells are implicated as contributors to the pathogenesis of many intestinal disease processes, including colitis and inflammatory bowel disease. Ginkgo, well known for its memory-enhancing effects, has potent antioxidant and anti-inflammatory activity. I have used ginkgo for cognitive, respiratory, and intestinal problems. In fact, I use ginkgo whenever more circulation is desired, regardless of the disease. Interestingly, ginkgo has been specifically studied in small intestinal ischemic injury and was found to provide protective effects against oxidative damage and intestinal permeability.[10] Ginkgo is one of the most versatile herbs that I have used. I prefer to use ginkgo phytosome for better absorption.

Fructo-Oligosaccharides (FOS)
Fructo-oligosaccharides are composed of one molecule of sucrose and one to three molecules of fructose.[11] They are found in varying amounts in many foods including honey, burdock, rye, asparagus, Jerusalem artichokes, bananas, and oats. They may also be supplemented in capsule form in the diet. FOS are virtually indigestible in the gastrointestinal tract; however, they are easily utilized by "friendly bacteria" and thus increase their population. FOS should be supplemented along with probiotics to discourage the growth of pathogenic bacteria.

It is imperative to remember that immune modulation—and ultimately strengthening of the immune system—will cure this disease. My list of biological response modifiers certainly is a great place to start, but it is just the tip of the iceberg.

IRRITABLE BOWEL SYNDROME
Irritable bowel syndrome (IBS) is a disease of exclusion. When other diseases such as inflammatory, infectious, parasitic, or neoplastic are excluded, a presumptive diagnosis of IBS is diagnosed. A thorough diagnostic work-up is necessary before a diagnosis is made.

In humans, this disorder has been termed a spastic or nervous colon. This disorder involves the large bowel. Clinical signs in dogs with IBS include passage of small amounts of mucoid stool with or without dyschezia (painful defecation) and increased frequency of defecation. Stools may be soft, formed, or watery diarrhea. Intermittent bloating, nausea, vomiting, and abdominal pain may also be present. The colon is histologically (microscopically) normal with no inflammatory cell infiltrates as in inflammatory bowel disease. It is generally believed that nervousness contributes to irritable bowel syndrome. Some dogs will get a "nervous" diarrhea while boarding; others that are low on the pecking order in a multiple dog household may be prone to diarrhea. Psychological factors contribute to this perplexing syndrome.

The most commonly prescribed treatment is supplementation with dietary fiber. I prefer to add crushed flax seeds to the raw food diet. At times, mood-altering herbs such as kava kava, valerian root, and St. John's wort may be used for their calming effects. In humans, enteric-coated peppermint oil capsules have shown to reduce colonic spasm and pain.[12] Peppermint oil capsules appear to have a relaxing and soothing effect on the intestines and thus quell spasm and pain.

CONSTIPATION

Some people define constipation as colonic retention of feces, caused by absent, infrequent, or difficult defecation. Constipated patients have excessive straining; hard, dry stools; abdominal pain; bloating; and incomplete evacuation of feces. To adopt a successful treatment plan, the underlying cause must be diagnosed. Some possible causes may include colonic or rectal masses, perineal hernias, and rectal strictures, to name just a few. It also might be idiopathic or due to unknown causes. Our discussion will be limited to idiopathic (unknown) causes.

When no specific disease is present, constipation is most likely "functional," resulting from an interaction of factors that may encompass physical, dietary, and age-related factors.

Peristalsis, the progressive wave-like movement from circular contractions of smooth muscles, normally and involuntarily propels the contents of the colon toward the rectum. Motor activity of the gastrointestinal tract is controlled and coordinated by intestinal nerves, which receive input from the autonomic and central nervous systems. Disruption of autonomic stimulation to the colon may produce constipation with lowered motility, colonic dilation, decreased rectal tone, and impaired defecation. This may be due to a host of causes including spinal and sacral nerve damage. Nutritional deficiencies, which affect the nervous system, can be significant contributors, again caused by dead processed enzymeless food. Remember one important thing: there is no such thing as a 100 percent balanced processed food. Since we do not know all there is to know about nutrition, how can we produce a 100 percent balanced processed diet? The answer is: only "nature" can produce a 100 percent balanced diet.

Ingesting sufficient fluid, consuming adequate and varied amounts of dietary fiber, obtaining ample quantities of nutrients for gastrointestinal health and function, and supporting bowel bacterial balance are all necessary to create and maintain a healthy colon and normal bowel function. Liver and/or gallbladder congestion or dysfunction causes diminished biliary secretion, which affects both digestion and excretion and contributes to constipation.

When constipation exists, waste matter moves too slowly, more fluid is absorbed (resulting in small, hard, dry stools), and feces remain in the bowel longer, so it putrefies and becomes toxic. These toxins may be absorbed in the circulatory system and cause further pathology.

Initial therapy for constipation is usually dietary, with an emphasis on increasing dietary fiber intake. Fiber increases stool weight and frequency of defecation and decreases gastrointestinal transit time. The bulking effect of fiber on stool may be due to additional water retention, proliferation of colonic bacteria, and proper production of gasses in stool. Insufficient fiber in the diet is the most common cause of constipation. Dietary fiber absorbs water and fats, softens the stools, and makes them easier to pass.

Since high fiber foods contain innumerable vitamin complexes, minerals, phytochemicals, and other natural substances, researchers cannot say for certain that fiber alone is responsible for the benefits they observe when such foods are consumed. Whole natural raw unprocessed foods have a cooperative and synergistic effect on the whole body.

There are two basic types of fiber: soluble and insoluble. Soluble fibers lubricate the fecal matter and increase bulk, which make elimination easier. This type of fiber is abundant in prunes, flax seeds, oats, beans, barley, carrots, potatoes, apples, and psyllium. Insoluble fiber is found in whole wheat, brown rice, other unrefined whole grains, unprocessed vegetables, fruits, and seeds (sunflower, pumpkin, sesame, etc.). Both types of fiber aid in bowel regularity.

Fiber is nature's broom, increasing stool weight and the speed stool travels through the intestines. It decreases abdominal discomfort and increases stool frequency. Processed foods become only a mop, not a broom. Vegetables and fruits should be consumed raw or steamed; nuts and seeds should be eaten raw; grains and beans must be cooked because they possess enzyme inhibitors. Remember, grains may be used in small amounts in the diet (less than 10 percent). Grains are high in vitamins and minerals, especially vitamin E complex. Grains that have been used include whole wheat bulgar, kasha, stone-ground corn meal, brown and wild rice, millet, quinoa, amaranth, whole rye, and steel-cut oats. I prefer to add sprouted wheat grass, barley, and other sprouted grains, all of which are high in vitamins and enzymes.

Foods containing fats have a lubricating effect on the mucous membrane lining of the colon walls. Fat-soluble vitamins and unsaturated fatty acids are important to the gastrointestinal tract. Vitamin A complex, B complex, E complex, and unsaturated fatty acids (especially omega-3 fatty acids) are all beneficial. Foods rich in these fat-associated nutrients are often a source of mucilage (gum-like gels). For example, the 12 percent mucilage content of flax seeds makes them the best natural laxative. I use crushed flax seeds in most gastrointestinal tract diseases.

Natural stimulant laxatives such as aloe, cascara sagrado, senna, and rhubarb work by directly increasing intestinal motor activity. Though considered safe, I only use these stimulants on an as-needed basis for short-term periods of time. Be careful about using these stimulants long-term; they may cause local irritation or a lazy bowel.

Last but not least, exercise is important to promote normal flow of energy and move bowel contents along. With exercise, the abdomen is massaged, and circulation in the gastrointestinal area is increased. Constipation can result from a lack of tone in abdominal muscles; activity strengthens this all-important muscle.

INTESTINAL PARASITES

There are a host of intestinal parasites that infect both dogs and cats. Several even have the potential to be zoonotic (transmitted to humans from animals). Modern drugs have excellent efficacy and safety and should be administered by your veterinarian. Stay away from outdated and dangerous wormers sold over-the-counter, as their efficacy and safety are questionable.

LIVER DISEASES

Liver diseases are common in dogs and cats and are life threatening. In cats, mild elevations of liver enzymes are far more serious than in the canine species. The liver can be directly damaged by a variety of toxic and infectious agents as well as a number of metabolic, immune-mediated, or neoplastic problems, or it may be secondarily affected.

Diagnosis of liver disease can require complete blood panels, ultrasounds, and ultrasound-guided liver biopsy. However, proceed with caution when contemplating liver biopsy; this is not a totally benign procedure. Clinical signs vary and may include anorexia, lethargy, vomiting, diarrhea, icterus, abdominal pain dehydration, and central nervous signs (encephalopathy). History is important in determining the source of liver failure. It could be the dietary indiscretion of eating a plant or raiding the garbage. Too often, though, the source is undetermined.

Let's look at the liver, how it functions in health and disease, and what we can do to help it in the detoxification process.

The liver is truly a remarkable organ with multiple functions.

It is the largest organ in the body, located on the right side in the upper abdomen. The liver quietly does an extraordinary job in keeping us alive and healthy by metabolizing the food we eat. It breaks food down into useful parts and protects us from the damaging effects of the numerous toxic compounds that we are exposed to on a daily basis. There are many chemicals in the food and water that both humans and animals eat, and these must all be detoxified. If you or your pet is ingesting synthetic fractionated vitamins, then your liver and kidney both must work harder in ridding the body of these chemicals. For example, with ingestion of ascorbic acid, your urine becomes abnormally bright; no such thing occurs when ingesting oranges, cherries, red peppers, etc. Your body recognizes food as natural and does not try to rid the body of it. Nature has developed this over millions of years while synthetic vitamins produced in a test tube have been developed by chemists in the last fifty or sixty years and the body has not adapted to them. In fact, the body is no more adapted to synthetic vitamins than it is to any other drug (antibiotics, tranquilizers, etc.) The liver has an impressive restorative capability, and is the only organ that will regenerate itself when part of it is damaged. This regeneration capacity is one of the intriguing survival mechanisms of the body.

Our health to a large extent depends on a well-functioning liver. I am always amazed at all the functions the liver must perform: while being exposed to a tremendous amount of potential damage, the liver is responsible for a multitude of essential functions related to metabolism, filtration, bile production, detoxification, and immune function.

The metabolic functions of the liver are countless. The liver is intricately involved in carbohydrate, fat, and protein metabolism, in storage of vitamins and minerals, and in many essential physiological processes. For example, the liver helps control blood sugar levels and hormone levels. It synthesizes proteins (such as plasma albumin, fibrinogen, and most globulins), lipids, and lipoproteins (phospholipids, cholesterol) as well as bile acids that are excreted in the detoxification process.

Detoxification is an essential part of the body's metabolism, and the liver plays a key role in this process. Toxic chemicals, both of internal and external origin, are constantly bombarding the liver. Our normal everyday metabolic processes actually produce a wide range of toxins that need to be taken care of by neutralizing mechanisms in the liver. Nutritional deficiencies and imbalances (processed food) add to the production of toxins, as do many drugs (acetaminophen, phenobarbital, prednisone). Toxins increase the stress on the liver by requiring a strong detoxification capacity.

It is our external environment, however, that contributes the most to the load of toxins that the liver has to detoxify. The burden on the liver today is heavier than ever before in history. There are at least 60,000 toxic chemicals in the environment today. Toxic chemicals are found in the food we and our pets eat, in the water we drink, and in the air we breathe both outdoors and indoors. There is ample evidence today of a connection between chemical exposure and chronic health problems to conclude that herbicides, pesticides, household chemicals, food additives, etc. create a serious health problem.

So, what happens when the liver's detoxification system is overloaded? The answer is simple. When the liver cannot do its job, the toxins that we and our pets are exposed to accumulate in the body and make us sick in various ways. They damage many body functions, particularly the immune system, and cause many chronic health problems. An overburdened and undernourished liver is known to be a root cause of many chronic diseases.

The liver plays several roles in detoxification. It filters the blood to remove large toxins, synthesizes and secretes bile full of cholesterol and other fat-soluble toxins, and enzymaticly disassembles unwanted chemicals. This enzymatic process occurs in two steps referred to as Phase I and Phase II. Phase I chemically modifies the chemicals to make them an easier target for one or more of the several Phase II enzyme systems.

Having an effective detoxification system is imperative for the well-being of our pets. For example, many diseases, including cancer, autoimmune disorders, neurological disorders, and the impairment of the immune system seen with aging, have been shown to be linked to a poorly functioning liver detoxification system.[13]

Phase I enzymes directly neutralize some chemicals and convert others to intermediate forms that are then processed by Phase II enzymes. Unfortunately, these intermediate forms are often more chemically active and therefore more toxic, so if the Phase II detoxification systems are not working adequately, these intermediates linger around and are far more damaging.

Phase I detoxification of most toxins involves a group of enzymes called cytochrome P-450. Some fifty to one hundred enzymes make up the cytochrome P-450 system. Each enzyme works best in detoxifying certain types of chemicals, but with considerable overlap in activity among the enzymes. In other words, they all metabolize the same chemicals, but with differing levels of efficiency. Evolution has ensured maximum detoxification. However, if for some reason toxins impair the P-450 system, an individual becomes more susceptible to carcinogens and cancer.

When cytochrome P-450 metabolizes a toxin, it tries to either chemically transform it into a less toxic form, make it water-soluble, or convert it to a more chemically active form. Making a toxin water-soluble enables the kidney to excrete it in the urine. Transforming the toxin into a more chemically reactive form makes it more easily metabolized by Phase II enzymes. Though important to good health, this transformation into more chemically active toxins can cause problems.[14]

A significant side effect of all this metabolic activity is the production of free radicals as toxins are transformed. Without adequate antioxidants, every time the liver neutralizes a toxin, it is damaged by the free radicals produced.

This is how poisonous mushrooms or acetaminophen damage the liver: the liver produces so many free radicals while neutralizing the toxins that the liver cells are overwhelmed and destroyed in the process. The most important antioxidant for neutralizing the free radicals produced as Phase I by-products is the sulfur-containing antioxidant, glutathione. Glutathione is required for one of the Phase II detoxification processes. When high levels of toxin exposure produce so many free radicals from Phase I detoxification that all the glutathione is used up, Phase II glutathione conjugation stops working. This is what occurs when cats ingest acetaminophen. They lack an enzyme called glucuronyl transferase and so will produce enormous amounts of free radical activity, which eventually destroys the liver and kills the cat. Therefore, the rate at which Phase I produces activated intermediates must be balanced by the rate at which Phase II finishes their processing.

Phase II typically involves a process called conjugation, in which various enzymes in the liver attach small chemicals to the toxin. This either neutralizes it or makes it more easily excreted through the urine or bile. In short, Phase II enzymes act on some toxins directly, while others must first be activated by Phase I enzymes.

Some researchers believe there is a Phase III system called antiporter activity.[15] In this multi-drug resistance system, the small intestinal cells pump toxins out of the cells back into the intestinal lumen. This allows toxins to go through a Phase I detoxification again and decreases toxins within the small intestines. Remember, when treating liver disease, a nontoxic, unprocessed raw food diet must be implemented. Socrates once said, "Let food be your medicine and medicine be your food," or something to that effect. Anyway, we must minimize the ingestion of toxins and processed food (even if they have a natural sounding name). They will inhibit the healing process. Ingestion of "live" foods—not dead processed food—is for the living.

Artichoke
Artichoke extract has demonstrated a strong antioxidant potential and hepatoprotective (liver protecting) effect in recent research on animals.[16] It protects the liver and the animal from the

damaging effects of toxins, such as carbon tetrachloride and other environmental chemicals in a manner similar to that of silymarin from milk thistle. Like milk thistle, artichoke extract is also able to stimulate regeneration of damaged liver tissue.

Beets
Growing up as a child, I saw my parents frequently drink an Eastern European drink made from beets called borsch. My father said it helped his digestion. Well, it turns out he was correct; not only does it help digestion, but it is a great liver detoxifier. Betaine, a natural constituent of sugar beets, has actions similar to those of artichoke. Betaine acts on the methylation cycle in liver cells, functioning as a methyl donor. This has the potential to promote the regeneration of liver cells and transport fat out of the liver (lipolysis). This may have beneficial effects in fatty liver syndrome in obese cats. Beets contain phosphorus, sodium, magnesium, calcium, iron, potassium, fiber, vitamin C, carotenoids, niacin, folic acid, and biotin.

Brassica Family Foods (Cabbage, Broccoli, Brussels Sprouts)
The brassica family foods contain chemical constituents that stimulate both Phase I and Phase II detoxification enzymes. These foods are high in vitamin C and a chemical called indole-3-carbinol. Both of these nutrients have a synergistic effect in detoxifying the liver and cancer protection.

Curcumin
This Indian herb is a potent antioxidant and anti-inflammatory. Curcumin has been shown to have bile-secreting effects. Curcumin also possesses liver protective activity, detoxifies dangerous carcinogens, stimulates the gallbladder, and acts as a free-radical scavenger. It appears that curcumin exerts its anticarcinogenic activity by lowering the activation of carcinogens while increasing the detoxification (stimulating Phase II) of those that are activated.

N, N-Dimethylglycine (DMG)

Several amino acids (glycine being one of them) are used to combine with and neutralize toxins. It appears that glycine is the most commonly utilized in Phase II amino acid detoxification. Humans and animals suffering from hepatitis, liver disorders, carcinomas, chronic arthritis, hypothyroidism, and excessive chemical exposure are commonly found to have a poorly functioning amino acid conjugation system (Phase II). This means that in those with liver disease, all the toxins requiring this pathway stay in the body doing damage almost twice as long.[17]

N, N-Dimethylglycine is a tertiary amino acid and is a natural component of animal and plant metabolism. DMG is a normal physiologically active nutrient found in low levels in such foods as grains, seeds, liver, eggs, and other high protein foods. In the body, the liver converts DMG into other useful metabolites by a process known as oxidative demethylation.[18]

DMG supports transmethylation processes through its ability to give up its methyl groups to help produce sulfur-adenosylmethionine (SAMe). SAMe is the principle methyl donor in the body, and transmethylation involves the reaction whereby a methyl group (CH_3) is transferred from SAMe to another molecule. It is a biochemical process, which is essential to life, health, and regenerative processes. In short, the body detoxifies potentially damaging chemicals and regulates a number of cellular processes through SAMe.

DMG has also been shown to be a potent biological response modifier. It can strengthen the immune system while assisting the body in fighting against foreign antigens such as bacteria, viruses, and other pathogens.[19] This is a versatile nutrient that I have used successfully for both immune enhancement and treatment of liver disease.

D-Glucarate

As stated before, in Phase II reactions, a chemical actually attaches to the carcinogen or toxin in order to help eliminate it from the body. Phase II reactions are called conjugates. The primary purpose of this type of detoxification system is to rapidly convert dangerous chemicals to conjugated (bound) forms that are water-soluble and easily excreted from the body. One of the most important Phase II reactions in the body is the conjugation reaction that uses D-glucarate. D-glucarate helps the body remove carcinogens, toxins, and compounds that are no longer needed.[20] D-glucarate is found in fruits and vegetables and is also made in the body from glucose. It can also be ingested as a supplement. D-glucarate exhibits potent antioxidant activity.

Conjugation with glucuronic acid appears to be the principal conjugation pathway in the tissues of humans and all animals. This process is called glucuronidation. Glucuronidation appears to be an important mechanism for detoxification from compounds produced by the body and environmental toxins. This process is one of the major known detoxification pathways in tissues of all vertebrates.[21] Glucuronic acid and carcinogen or toxin binding occur primarily in the liver. The complex is picked up by bile (which contains waste products) and then is carried to the intestines, where it is removed in the feces. The complex can also pass through the kidneys to be excreted in the urine. Glucuronyl transferase is the enzyme that performs the conjugation reaction between toxins and glucuronic acid.

However, an enzyme called beta-glucuronidase often throws a monkey wrench into the works. Remember that enzymes are proteins that speed up chemical reactions. Many chemical reactions are reversible, which means the products can change back into toxic-starting materials. In this case, beta-glucuronidase reverses the conjugation of compounds that are bound to glucuronic acid, allowing them to go free and cause damage. Thus, beta-glucuronidase can be considered a bad enzyme because it reverses the process that rids the body of toxins or carcinogens.

But the body still has more tricks up its sleeve in the detoxification process. Active sites on enzymes are special locations where chemical reactions are sped up. The compound that is getting chemically altered or changed is called the substrate. The substrate must bind to this active site in order for the reaction to occur. Because enzymes have specificity, there is usually only one substrate that gets altered chemically. Here is the good news: sometimes a different compound, one that is not altered, goes into the active site. When this happens, the substrate cannot react with the enzyme. It has been shown D-glucarate binds to the active site of beta-glucuronidase thus inhibiting the reversal of conjugation, allowing toxins to be eliminated from the body. This is good because it happens even in the presence of beta-glucuronidase (bad enzyme), because the D-glucurate stops deconjugation (allowing detoxification).

Scientists found that D-glucarate can go through enzymatic reactions and produce a substance called D-glucaro-1,4-lactone (GL). It was found that GL was the active substance involved in the inhibition of beta-glucuronidase. The related compound, D-glucaric acid, is found in foods such as apples, grapefruits, and brassica family foods (broccoli). D-glucarate can also be produced in the body from glucuronic acid. D-glucaric acid can be converted to GL in the body.

As D-glucaric acid enters the body, it is absorbed in the gastrointestinal tract and maintained in the bloodstream. It is then transported in the blood to various organs to help in detoxification and is eventually excreted in the bile or urine.

It was found that calcium D-glucarate will increase the level of GL in the body.

Essentially, the body benefits from increased detoxification primarily in the liver.

Glutathione

A primary detoxification route is the conjugation of glutathione (composed of cystein, glutamic acid, and glycine). The liver enzyme glutathione s-transferase takes sulfur from glutathione and combines it with toxic substances, making it water-soluble. This water-soluble form is then easily excreted in the urine. The best natural sources of glutathione precursors are eggs and raw milk. I also use a stabilized glutathione product, which further increases blood glutathione levels.

Glutathione is an important neutralizer of free radicals produced when the liver neutralizes toxins through the Phase I pathway. Glutathione appears to be especially important in organs exposed to toxins, such as the liver, kidneys, lungs, and intestines. It also supports Phase II detoxification.

I use stabilized glutathione in the treatment of practically all diseases since it is a potent and versatile detoxifier, free radical scavenger, and immune enhancer.

Licorice

Licorice exerts many actions that are beneficial in acute and chronic liver disease including: protecting the liver, enhancing the immune system, potentiating interferon, working as the body's own antiviral and immune-enhancing agent, and promoting the flow of bile and fat to and from the liver.[22]

Glycyrrhiza has been shown to have a direct hepatoprotective effect. The primary hepatoprotective constituent is the triterpene glycoside, glycyrrhizin (also known as glycyrrhetinic acid). This flavonoid has been shown to protect hepatocytes exposed to carbon tetrachloride.[23] It appears that a major protective mechanism is its antilipid peroxidation as well as potent free radical quenching effects.

Recent studies have also shown that licorice has the ability to enhance detoxification of drugs and toxins. Increased liver glucuronidation is one mechanism of detoxification. Rats pretreated with a glycyrrhiza tincture significantly increased the cumulative biliary and urinary excretion of acetaminophen-glucuronide conjugate within 120 minutes after the administration of acetaminophen.[24] I usually use licorice for only six to eight weeks at a time; prolonged use may produce hypertension.

Liver Extracts

The oral administration of hydrolyzed liver extracts has been used in the treatment of liver disease for many years. Recent scientific investigations into the therapeutic efficacy of liver extracts have demonstrated that these extracts promote hepatic regeneration and are quite effective in the treatment of chronic liver disease including hepatitis.[25]

Milk Thistle (Silybum Marianum)

Milk thistle has been used for centuries as an herbal medicine for the treatment of liver disease. The active constituent in milk thistle is silymarin, a mixture of three flavolignans. Silybin is the most biologically active flavonoid in silymarin.

Therapeutically, milk thistle acts by protecting liver cells from toxic damage,[26] boosting glutathione concentrations,[27] and regenerating normal liver cells.[28] Milk thistle is also a potent free radical scavenger. In humans, milk thistle has been used clinically for a number of conditions including alcoholic liver disease, hepatitis, amanita mushroom poisoning, and skin disease. Silymarin has also shown to enhance liver detoxification by inhibition of Phase I detoxification while enhancing glucuronidation.[29] One of the most important aspects of this herb is that it slows down or even reverses the formation of fibrosis (scar tissue) in the liver.[30] This is my main herbal treatment in liver disease.

Picrorhiza Kurroa

Picrorhiza is an important herb in the traditional Ayurvedic system of medicine and has been used to treat liver disease and bronchial problems. The most important active constituents of picrorhiza are the iridoid glycosides known collectively as kutkin.[31] Like silymarin, picrorhiza possesses significant antioxidant activity, which in part contributes to its hepatoprotective ability. It was found that picrorhiza restored depleted glutathione levels in African desert rats infected with malaria.[32]

Like silymarin, picrorhiza may have an effect on liver

regeneration. A 1992 study demonstrated that picrorhiza has comparable liver regenerative abilities to silymarin.[33]

Picrorhiza has been shown to possess potent anti-inflammatory ability, which may at least in part contribute to its hepatoprotective effects. Apocynin, one of its constituents, has been shown to be responsible for its anti-inflammatory effects.[34] I have used this versatile herb for both liver disease and immune suppressed animals. However, picrorhiza has been shown to have at least as potent hepatoprotective effects as silymarin.[35] It has been used in amanita mushroom poisoning, aflatoxin B (fungus), and carbon tetrachloride (liver toxin) experiments with impressive results.[36]

Perhaps picrorhiza's hepatoprotective effects are due to its potent choleretic (bile stimulating) effects. In fact, silymarin was tested simultaneously for comparison and was found to have weaker choleretic effects.[37] By quickly ridding the body of toxins through bile stimulation, the body is detoxified much faster and thus healing ensues.

This herb is bitter, and there may be difficulties in administering it to cats. However, it can easily be administered to dogs with food.

Phosphatidylcholine (PC)
Phosphatidycholine (PC), the main component of lecithin, is a phospholipid, a kind of fat that is found throughout the body as an integral part of cell membranes. It is essential for their structural and functional integrity. Cell membranes act like gatekeepers, allowing nutrients into the cells while blocking toxins from entering the cell. Supplemental PC from soybean extracts has been shown to enhance the functional integrity of cell membranes.

Although it has not been clearly established how PC exerts its protective effect, it is believed that it has something to do with its ability to be incorporated into normal and damaged liver cell membranes. When PC is incorporated into cell membranes, it is believed that this increases membrane fluidity and thus the

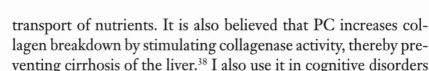

transport of nutrients. It is also believed that PC increases collagen breakdown by stimulating collagenase activity, thereby preventing cirrhosis of the liver.[38] I also use it in cognitive disorders as well.

S-Adenosylmethionine (SAMe)

S-Adenosylmethionine (SAMe) is an important physiological agent formed in the body by combining the essential amino acid methionine with adenosyl-triphosphate (ATP). Normally the body manufactures all the SAMe it needs from methionine, as long as there is ample vitamin B_{12} or folic acid available. SAMe is probably the most important methyl donor in methylation reactions and is important in more than forty biochemical reactions in the body.[39]

In humans, supplementation with SAMe for patients with liver cirrhosis results in not only improved bile flow but also improved membrane function and increased levels of glutathione.[40, 41] Improved membrane fluidity presumably helps in minimizing cirrhosis and scar tissue in the liver, thus improving bile flow and circulation in the liver.

chapter 10

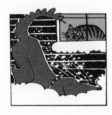

Endocrine Diseases: Combining Holistic and Traditional Methods

IN THIS CHAPTER, WE WILL LOOK AT SOME HORMONALLY RELATED DISEASES, and what we can do to alleviate or cure these problems. As a "holistic" oriented veterinarian, I use all of the arsenals at my disposal. This means I integrate the best that modern science has to offer along with complementary modalities—I use both herbs and modern medicines. Truly, a holistic doctor must use all that will help the patient, no matter where the help comes from. Nature has given us many medicines to date and, in the future, will give us many more; until then, we should use man's modern research and ingenuity to heal both humans and animals alike.

DIABETES INSIPIDUS

Diabetes insipidus (DI) is caused by the deficiency of antidiuretic hormone or the lack of response by the kidneys to this hormone. This hormone (antidiuretic) is produced by the posterior pituitary, which signals the kidneys to concentrate the urine. The most common signs seen are polyuria (increased urine) and polydipsia (increased drinking). Many other diseases produce symptoms similar to DI: diabetes mellitus, Cushing's syndrome, liver disease, kidney disease, cystitis (bladder infection), and even psychogenic problems.

A thorough blood panel and urinalysis must be instituted to rule out other disorders. Urinalysis frequently reveals a specific gravity (urine concentration) of less than 1.010 consistently. This is a dilute urine; healthy urine should be at least 1.025 specific gravity concentration. Frequently, serial urinalysis must be performed to diagnose this problem.

This disease is caused by either a lesion or trauma to the brain or insensitivity of the kidneys to antidiuretic hormone. The standard treatment for this disease is DDAVP (desmopressin). There are two forms of this drug: One form is an intranasal spray that is used by placing one or two drops in alternating eyes (conjunctival sac). The other form is 0.1 mg tablets. I dose at ¼ to 1 tablet once or twice daily to effect, depending on size. Both forms of desmopressin are expensive; however, there is much less waste with the tablet form, which I prefer to use. Desmopressin is safe and effective and should be used in the treatment of DI.

DIABETES MELLITUS

Diabetes mellitus (DM) is a complex endocrine disorder, which occurs when the pancreas stops producing the hormone insulin or the body becomes unable to use the insulin it produces. The most common clinical signs observed are increased drinking and urination. I see this disease more frequently in cats than dogs. In humans, it is thought to be caused by an autoimmune disease. I believe that in pets DM is caused in susceptible individuals by processed, dead, and enzymeless foods, which over time overtax the pancreas causing an inflammatory response.

As excessive glucose in the blood spills over into the urine, electrolytes are lost, and dehydration and muscle wasting is observed. These pets are also susceptible to cystitis (bladder infection). It has also been found that high blood sugar levels in diabetics tend to block the delta-6-desaturase enzyme resulting in decreased production of anti-inflammatory prostaglandins.[1] This may result in increased pruritis (itching) in atopic patients as well as neurologic or eyesight problems. I prefer to administer crushed flax seeds, which are high in omega-3 fatty acids and offer anti-inflammatory properties as well as high fiber content.

This is a life-threatening disease. If your pet has DM, it should be under the care of a veterinarian. It is important that the veterinarian and pet guardian work closely together using insulin injection, diet, and complementary therapies to benefit the patient. I prefer to use PZI insulin on a once daily injection regime. At least fifty percent of my patients no longer needed insulin after several months of treatments.

Diet should be restricted to a natural raw food diet with the phasing out of all processed foods. As I mentioned previously, I prefer to administer crushed flax seeds for its soluble fiber content. In fact, it has been shown that adding high fiber in the form of psyllium to diabetic men decreased both blood glucose and lipids.[2] It is imperative to feed a raw food diet to decrease inflammation in the pancreas while allowing it to heal. Feeding mainly raw meat, eggs, some vegetables, and nutritional yeast lowers blood glucose. If available, raw milk provides an array of life-giving nutrients. Do not feed grains, as it may exacerbate the problem.

In the future, pancreas transplantation will be commonplace to replace insulin injections. There is also ongoing research into oral administration of insulin. The following remedies have been used in diabetics.

Alpha Lipoic Acid

Alpha lipoic acid can be synthesized by both animals and humans.[3] Unfortunately, we manufacture only enough of the nutrient to prevent a deficiency. That is not enough for the nutrient to live up to its full potential, thus we need to eat food rich in lipoic acid such as potatoes, yeast, liver, carrots, beets, and especially red meat or take supplementation.

Lipoic acid is a sulfur-containing compound and plays a vital role as the critical cofactor in the fundamental production of cellular energy. First, lipoic acid aids in the conversion of carbohydrates into energy. During the metabolizing process of blood sugar into energy, the sugar is transformed into pyruvic acid. Pyruvic acid is a product of a process called glycolysis, which is the first step in converting blood sugar into energy that the body can burn. This metabolic activity of lipoic acid occurs inside the cells, within the mitochondria. Mitochondria are often referred to as the "engine" of the cell, where food is converted into energy.

Lipoic acid not only improves metabolism, it also protects the body against harmful by-products of metabolism. It does so by attaching to and preventing the oxidation of certain enzymes during the metabolic process. This act of binding to enzymes not only protects the enzymes from oxidation, but allows them to be used by the body again and again, rather than becoming waste material.

Chemical reactions occur in the body by the thousands every second. During these reactions, electrons are continuously shifted around from one place and task to another, removing toxins and waste, fighting infections, breathing, walking, etc. All of these chemical reactions cause free radical reactions. This is where the versatile alpha lipoic acid shines as a nutrient.

Though a relatively new antioxidant in the United States, alpha lipoic acid has been used in Germany for more than thirty years. Alpha lipoic acid is an important broad-spectrum antioxidant able to quench a wide range of free radicals in both water and lipid (fat) environments. Moreover, it has the remarkable ability to recycle several other important antioxidants including vitamins C and E, glutathione, and coenzyme Q_{10}, as well as itself. This is truly a universal antioxidant.

Alpha lipoic acid helps diabetics normalize blood sugar levels. Research has shown that it protects rat pancreatic islet cells from free radical damage.[4] It was also found to stimulate glucose uptake by muscle cells in a manner similar to insulin.[5] In a placebo-controlled human study, it was demonstrated that alpha lipoic acid increased insulin sensitivity and thus enhanced glucose uptake in Type II diabetics (noninsulin-dependent diabetics).[6]

Coenzyme Q_{10}

Studies have shown that diabetics have depressed levels of coenzyme Q_{10}, especially insulin-dependent diabetics.[7] Interestingly, coenzyme Q_{10} has shown both protective effects and improved beta cell function and glycemic control in Type II or noninsulin-dependent diabetics.[8]

Figure 10.1
COQ_{10} Tissue Concentrations

ORGAN	MCG/GRAM
Heart	114.0
Kidney	66.5
Liver	54.9
Pancreas	32.7
Brain	13.4
Colon	10.7

Source: Beth M. Lay Jacobs, Ph.D., 1999[9]

As can be seen, the pancreas requires a high concentration of coenzyme Q_{10}. Only the heart, kidney, and liver possess more coenzyme Q_{10}.

Fenugreek

Fenugreek has been studied, particularly in India, for the treatment of diabetes. Fenugreek seeds contain an alkaloid constituent known as trigonelline, which is thought to be responsible for at least some of fenugreek's action on reducing hyperglycemia. Fenugreek also contains nicotinic acid, coumarins, and saponins, all compounds known to have important physiologic effects. Nicotinic acid has been shown to inhibit insulinase, the enzyme that breaks down insulin in humans.[10] Fenugreek extracts were also observed to reduce post-prandial (after eating) serum glucose, glucagon, insulin, cholesterol, and triglycerides in both normal and diabetic test dogs.[11]

Vitamin C and Bioflavonoids

There are well-known complications in diabetics such as cataracts, retinopathy, nephropathy, and neuropathy, just to name a few. Much of this is due to the "sorbitol pathway." This pathway converts glucose to sorbitol and then to fructose. It is especially active in diabetics as glucose rises in tissues that are not insulin sensitive (lens of eye, kidneys, peripheral nerves). It is a bit technical, but is important to understand in order to give diabetics all that will improve their lives. Excess glucose passively diffuses into cells and is reduced to sorbitol by nicotinamide adenine dinacleotide phosphate (NADPH) with the help of an enzyme known as aldose reductase. In the presence of NADPH, sorbitol is oxidized to fructose, catalyzed by the enzyme sorbitol dehydrogenase. Since sorbitol does not diffuse passively through cell membranes, it accumulates, along with some fructose within the cell, thus resulting in cell damage. If we can inhibit the enzyme aldose reductose, then we can prevent glucose from being reduced to sorbitol.

There are many natural and safe aldose reductase inhibitors (ARIs). Among the most prominent are vitamin C and various bioflavonoids such as quercetin, naringin, and hesperidin.[12] It is obvious that ARIs prevent complications in the diabetic patient. Quercitin appears to be the most potent physiologically active bioflavonoid. Remember, natural vitamin C (not ascorbic acid) is in part composed of bioflavonoids.

Glucose Tolerance Factor (GTF)

Foods rich in glucose tolerance factor (GTF) include nutritional yeast, liver, whole grains, eggs, buckwheat, mushrooms, beets, prunes, nuts, and potatoes with skin. In fact, most fresh foods in their natural state are a good source of dietary chromium complexes. Nutritional yeast has been shown to be the highest source of GTF. Refined and processed foods may have as much as 80 percent of their naturally occurring chromium removed.

GTF along with insulin make it easier for carbohydrates, fatty acids, and amino acids to pass from the blood into the cells of various tissues. It also promotes the metabolism of nutrients within the cells. When GTF is lacking, more insulin is needed to perform these jobs. In its biologically active form (natural foods), chromium is part of the hormone-like GTF; it functions primarily as an insulin cofactor.[13] GTF aids insulin's ability to transport glucose and amino acids inside cells for energy and tissue production. Deficiency has been shown to lead to insulin resistance (inability to utilize insulin).

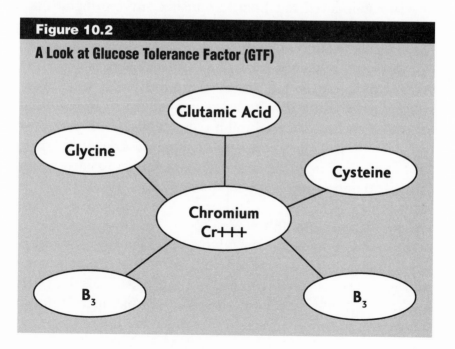

Figure 10.2

A Look at Glucose Tolerance Factor (GTF)

As you can see GTF is a trivalent chromium surrounded by two molecules of B_3 (niacinamide) and three amino acids of glycine, glutamic acid, and cysteine. Remember, these three amino acids make up glutathione, probably the most important antioxidant in the body.

Unfortunately, modern widespread agricultural practices have led to widespread chromium deficits in the food supply. Buying organically grown foods will help with higher nutrient levels in our foods. Feeding a natural raw food diet will prevent diabetes, and starting pets off at an early age on a natural food diet will prevent many other degenerative diseases as well.

Gymnema Sylvestre

Gymnema sylvestre, a plant native to India, has been used for the treatment of diabetes for more than 2,000 years. It has been found to increase urine output and reduce hyperglycemia in both animal and human studies. Gymnema's antidiabetic activity appears to be due to a combination of mechanisms. Two animal studies on diabetic-induced rats found gymnema extracts doubled the number of insulin-secreting beta cells in the pancreas and returned blood sugars to almost normal.[14, 15]

In a controlled study, a standardized extract was given to twenty-seven Type I diabetic humans for six to thirty months. Thirty-seven others continued on insulin therapy alone and were treated for ten to twelve months. Insulin requirements were decreased by about one-half and the average blood glucose decreased from 232 mg/dl to 152 mg/dl in the gymnema group. The control group showed no improvement during the study.[16]

Momordica Charantia (Bitter Melon)

Bitter melon is found in China, India, Asia, and Africa, where it has a historical use for diabetes. The active hypoglycemic constituents include charantin and a polypeptide called p-insulin (plant insulin). This polypeptide is structurally and pharmacologically comparable to bovine insulin.[17] Several studies in both humans and animals have confirmed the blood sugar lowering effects of momordica extracts.[18, 19] As its name implies, this is a bitter fruit; however, it is now available in capsule form, which makes it convenient and acceptable to both humans and pets alike.

Vaccinium Myrtillus (Bilberry)

Bilberry has traditionally been used to improve eyesight and inhibit cataract formation. However, its biologically active constituents known as anthocyanosides also have blood sugar lowering effects. In a study of diabetic-induced rats, plasma glucose was reduced by 26 percent.[20] One important attribute of bilberry is its ability to stabilize collagen.[21] Bilberry has been shown to decrease abnormal collagen formation and capillary permeability, thus helping to prevent retinopathy. Bilberry's beneficial effects are not restricted to the eyes, and it should be used whenever capillary stabilization is desired. I have prevented the formation of cataracts with the administration of bilberry.

Vanadium

Vanadium is a trace mineral that lowers blood sugar by mimicking insulin and improving cell sensitivity to insulin. This interesting trace mineral affects many aspects of carbohydrate metabolism such as glucose transport, breakdown of glucose, glucose output, sugar-processing enzymes, decrease of storage sugar production, and increased deposition. However, if given as an isolated mineral, it causes vomiting and nausea, particularly in cats. As with other nutrients, it is normally found in foods that are rich in vitamin E, so there must be a synergistic effect. Good natural sources include seafood, liver, whole grains, mushrooms, parsley, corn, and dill.

Zinc Rich Foods

Zinc is involved in virtually all aspects of insulin metabolism. Zinc also has a protective effect against beta cell destruction and possibly antiviral effects. Diabetics typically excrete excessive amounts of zinc in the urine and therefore require a zinc rich diet, which will improve insulin levels.[22, 23] Good sources are whole grains, oysters, beef, dark meat turkey, leek, legumes, seeds, nuts, crab, sardines, various fish, tuna, cheese, mustard greens, and fermented soy products.

HYPERADRENOCORTICISM (CUSHING'S SYNDROME)

Hyperadrenocorticism most commonly occurs due to excessive adrenocorticotrophic hormone (ACTH) output from the pituitary gland or overproduction of cortisol by an adrenocortical tumor. It may also be caused by the administration of pharmacological doses of glucocorticoids. These are dogs with chronic pruritic (itching) problems of the skin. This is termed iatrogenic (man-made) Cushing's syndrome.

Clinical signs are slow to develop and may include polyuria (increased urination), polydipsia (increased thirst), polyphagia (increased appetite), obesity, pot-bellied appearance, lethargy, thinning skin and hair, and bilateral symmetrical alopecia (loss of hair).

Diagnosis is confirmed with a thorough blood work-up, ACTH stimulation, and urinalysis. There may be secondary problems such as diabetes mellitus, infections, liver disease, pancreatitis, and severe immunosuppression. With the iatrogenic patient, I am usually able to "wean" them off of the glucocorticoids within six to eight weeks while building their immune systems and treating other problems such as liver disease or diabetes mellitus. These patients must be on a natural raw food diet, biological response modifiers, and a detoxification program. With a little work and patience, these dogs will do well.

Eighty-five percent of Cushing's syndrome in dogs is found to be the pituitary dependent variety. Most of these patients have a pituitary adenoma tumor producing excessive amounts of ACTH.

Standard allopathic therapy involves the use of lysodren, which targets the adrenal gland for destruction. This drug is powerful and effective in decreasing the production of cortisol. However, it also destroys the minerolocorticoid-producing area of the adrenal gland. In the hands of an experienced practitioner, this drug can alleviate the symptoms of hyperadrenocortism. Blood testing at seven- to fourteen-day intervals is required initially to assess treatment. If animals are hypothyroid or are depressed due to low cortisol or mineralocorticoid levels, then these conditions also must be addressed.

Ketoconozole, an antifungal drug, though safer than lysodren, is much less effective in decreasing cortisol production by the adrenal glands. This drug has the potential to produce hepatopathy in some patients. Selegiline has also been used with mixed results.

Unfortunately, there are no complementary treatments at this time that will produce adrenal gland destruction as lysodren has been shown to do. Complementary treatments are an adjunct to the use of lysodren. This is a life-threatening condition, and therefore, close and careful treatment and monitoring must be instituted at all times. DHEA, a precursor to adrenal hormones, may reduce the side effects of high blood cortisol levels.

HYPOADRENOCORTICISM (ADDISON'S DISEASE)

Before discussing hypoadrenocorticism or Addison's disease, we should discuss what the adrenals do under normal homeostatic conditions. We have already seen that Cushing's syndrome is life threatening from an overactive adrenal gland. Hypoadrenocorticism also is life threatening, if not treated correctly, for just the opposite: it is an adrenal deficiency.

The adrenals are two relatively crescent-shaped glands that are found lying over the upper pole of each kidney. Each adrenal gland consists of internal layers that produce different substances. The inner part, or adrenal medulla, manufactures epinephrine and norepinephrine, more commonly known as adrenaline and noradrenaline. These hormones are the "fight or flight" hormones that are released in potentially "life or death" situations. Their release increases heart rate and blood pressure and diverts more blood to the brain, heart, and skeletal muscles. This is important when dealing with stress or adrenal insufficiency (Addison's disease).

The adrenal cortex lies outside the adrenal medulla and responds to a different type of stress. This is where the steroid hormones are produced. They include cortisone, hydrocortisone, testosterone, estrogen, 17-hydroxy-ketosteroids, DHEA, DHEA sulfate, pregnenalone, aldosterone, androstenedione, progesterone, and some other hormones. Many of these hormones are made elsewhere in the body, but aldosterone, cortisone, and hydrocortisone are made only in the adrenal glands.

The hormone aldosterone, in concert with the kidneys, regulates the balance of sodium and potassium in the body. This regulation is critical to many areas of physiological function, including the ability to react to stress and to maintain fluid balance. It even contributes to maintenance of blood pressure.

In dogs, with primary hypoadrenocorticism, destruction of the adrenal glands leads to decreased production of glucocorticoids, mineralocorticoids, or both. In dogs with secondary disease, decreased secretion of corticotropin (ACTH) by the pituitary or corticotropin-releasing hormone (CRH) by the hypothalamus leads to decreased production of glucocorticoids.[24]

Clinical signs may mimic many other diseases and can only be confirmed with blood tests. I prefer the ACTH stimulation test. Signs may include lethargy, vomiting, anorexia, weakness, depression, diarrhea, dehydration, and in severe cases, collapse and shock.

Usually, the cause of adrenal failure cannot be identified; therefore, primary hypoadrenocorticism is usually classified as idiopathic (unknown). However, I believe this disease is due to an immune-mediated destruction of the adrenal glands. Interestingly, most of these patients are also hypothyroid, a known autoimmune disease.[25] Long-term allopathic maintenance treatment for Addison's disease consists of supplementation with mineralcorticoid (FLORINEF) and glucocorticoid (cortisone or hydrocortisone). [26]

Successful treatment must include a natural raw food diet supplemented with Celtic Sea Salt™ and kelp, as these are high in trace elements and minerals. Since the adrenal glands are high in vitamin C, fruits and vegetables to taste must be added to the diet. Remember, ascorbic acid is not vitamin C but only a small fractional part of it. Eskimos get their vitamin C from eating the adrenal glands of seals and thus prevent scurvy. Ascorbic acid will not cure scurvy.

Licorice, a sweet herb, reduces the amount of hydrocortisone broken down by the liver, thereby reducing the workload on the adrenal glands. Some patients may respond to adrenal cortical extracts (glandular product). Adrenal extracts are made from the whole adrenal gland or from just the adrenal cortex. The whole extract contains all of the hormones in their proper proportions and may be used safely and effectively. Panax ginseng, the most potent of all the adaptogenic herbs, has the ability to support and enhance the adrenal glands. Ginseng maximizes the use of oxygen and glycogen by working muscles, allowing them to function in an aerobic state for longer periods of time. Ginseng also helps the body maintain normal blood pressure and blood glucose levels. DHEA may also be used in this disease.

FELINE HYPERTHYROIDISM

Hyperthyroidism, or excessive concentrations of the circulating thyroid hormones, is now recognized as the most common endocrine disorder in cats.[27] The thyroid gland lies in the mid-portion of the neck and is easily palpated when enlarged. The thyroid gland secretes hormones that control the body's metabolic rate in two primary ways: by stimulating tissue response in the body to produce proteins and by increasing cell oxygenation. To produce these vital hormones, the thyroid needs the element iodine, which is ingested from food.

The regulation of thyroid hormone levels is controlled by several mechanisms. The hypothalamus, located in the brain just above the pituitary gland, secretes thyrotropin-releasing hormone, which triggers the pituitary to release thyroid-stimulating hormone (TSH). When the amount of thyroid hormone in the blood reaches a certain level, the pituitary will produce less thyroid-stimulating hormone; conversely, when the amount of thyroid hormone in the blood decreases to a certain level, the pituitary produces more thyroid-stimulating hormone.

There are two forms of thyroid hormones. Thyroxine (T_4), produced in the thyroid, has only a slight impact on speeding up the body's metabolic rate. Thyroxine is converted by the liver and other organs to triiodothyronine (T_3), which is the metabolically active form. Most of T_4 and T_3 remain tightly bound to certain proteins in the blood and in an inactive form. The body's continually changing need for more or less thyroid hormone will determine the rate of T_4 to T_3 conversion and the release of bound T_3 and T_4 in blood protein. In this way, the body will maintain the proper levels of thyroid hormone to regulate normal metabolic rate.

Feline hyperthyroidism is almost always due to a benign tumor of the thyroid gland, secreting excessive amounts of thyroid hormone. Since the majority of hyperthyroid cats are over ten years of age, I believe that these are slow-growing tumors, which take years to develop until clinical signs are finally observed.

As with all diseases, prevention is the best medicine. I believe that a combination of long-term ingestion of toxins in food and water, along with a low level of iodine in the food, causes feline hyperthyroidism. For example, chlorine and sodium fluoride added to municipal water supplies, chlorine-based chemicals found in bleaches, pesticides, and other products all promote thyroid disruption. Chlorine and fluoride may block iodine receptor sites on the thyroid, making it difficult or impossible for the gland to receive and utilize iodine.[28] This is why I recommend bottled or filtered water.

As previously stated, there are more than 60,000 chemicals in the environment, many with the potential to cause cancer of the thyroid gland. The list includes polybrominated biphenyls, polyhalogenated aromatic hydrocarbons, DDT, DDE, dieldrin and other organo-chlorines, PCBs, PBBs, and many more. Many petroleum and coal tar derivatives have the potential to cause thyroid tumors. These toxic compounds may appear in tap water, processed foods, pharmaceuticals, textiles, home furnishings, resins, adhesives, rubber products, plastic of all types, pesticides, herbicides, construction material, carpeting, and many other items. Red dye No. 3, popularly used in foods, cosmetics, and medications, was shown to consistently decrease T_3 levels, and increase T_4 and TSH levels.[29] Chronic inflammatory response in the thyroid gland along with toxins will cause thyroid adenoma and hyperthyroidism. It may be possible that the constant chemical barrage on the thyroid gland causes the gland to hypertrophy (enlarge) as a compensatory response—for example, to rectify an imbalance due to an iodine deficiency. The demands made upon the thyroid to produce its hormone without an adequate iodine supply result in hypertrophy (enlargement), which eventually becomes hyperplasia (excessive proliferation of normal cells) and eventually after long-term insult and inflammation becomes an adenomatous growth (tumor).

This disease is easily diagnosed with clinical signs and blood testing. Clinical signs may include vomiting, ravenous appetite and yet emaciation, dehydration, pacing, increased heart rate, and loss of muscle.

Most veterinarians treat hyperthyroidism with drugs such as tapazole, surgery, or radioactive iodine. Surgical excision carries the highest complication rate. Tapazole is relatively safe and considered the antithyroid drug of choice, but it may present some complications such as liver disease and anemia. Radioactive iodine, though expensive, may have the best cure rate. Unfortunately, complementary treatments have not been shown to be effective for this problem at this time.

Prevention offers the best medicine for our feline friends. A natural raw food diet supplemented with Celtic Sea Salt™ and/or kelp will provide vital nutrients including iodine for a healthy thyroid gland. Bottled or filtered drinking water should be offered at all times. Limitation of processed (canned or bagged) food devoid of enzymes and vital minerals will help prevent this problem.

CANINE HYPOTHYROIDISM

Canine hypothyroidism is the most common hormonal abnormality in the dog and is almost nonexistent in the cat. This condition is the result of reduced thyroid hormone secretion by the thyroid glands. The common symptoms of low thyroid function include chronic skin and haircoat problems, weight gain, lethargy, fatigue, depression, chronic infections, anemia, reproductive disorders, chronic otitis (ear infections), and musculoskeletal disorders.

In veterinary medicine, the most accurate diagnostic blood test is a free T_4 by equilibrium dialysis.[30] However, I have observed animals with normal blood tests that still exhibited signs of hypothyroidism. The form that affects the cells the most is T_3 (triiodothyronine), which is converted in the liver and other tissues from T_4. Thus, a dog can have a normal level of thyroid hormone in the blood, yet be thyroid deficient if the cells are not able to convert it to a more active T_3.

The most common cause is canine autoimmune thyroiditis. Genetics may certainly play a role since golden retrievers have the highest prevalence, followed by Shetland sheepdogs, cocker spaniels, boxers, Doberman pinschers, Labrador retrievers, Akitas, Irish setters, and English setters as the top ten breeds.[31]

The thyroid gland provides primary control of the rate of our metabolic activity. Apparently this control of metabolic rate is exerted through the impact of thyroid hormones on the mitochondria, the energy-generating organelles within our cells. In general, the higher the amount of thyroid hormone, the greater the number, size, and energy production of mitochondria. Thyroid hormones also have a great impact on how quickly molecules are transported across the cell membranes.

In addition to controlling the metabolic rate, the thyroid has a direct impact on the rate at which humans and animals grow and metabolize carbohydrates and fats. Blood tests routinely show a high cholesterol level in hypothyroid dogs.

Treatment of canine hypothyroidism includes a thyroid replacement product plus a high quality kelp product. Several nutrients are important to both the thyroid gland and the conversion of T_4 to the more active T_3. Some foods called goitrogens may have the ability to induce an iodine deficiency by combining with iodine and making it unavailable to the thyroid gland. Probably the worst offender is the soybean. Though championed as a health food, when eaten in excess, it may cause undesirable side effects. There are three "antinutrients" that soybeans may contain:

1. A large amount of phytic acid, which binds up and prevents absorption of minerals, especially zinc, calcium, and magnesium needed by the body.

2. Trypsin inhibitors, which cannot be refined out of the soy (trypsin is an important enzyme in digestion).

3. Isoflavones, genistein, and deidzein, three phytochemicals that have been shown to have antithyroid activity.[32] The soy isoflavones and other chemicals inhibit thyroid peroxidase, a key thyroid enzyme.

If you are thinking that this might be a good treatment for feline hyperthyroidism, it is unlikely that cats will ingest enough soy protein to be of benefit; however, research in this area might prove interesting. Unfortunately, the inhibition of thyroid peroxidase-catalyzed reactions results in decreased levels of circulating thyroid hormones, which lead to increased secretion of TSH by the anterior pituitary. The increased level of TSH provides a growth stimulus to the thyroid, and it has been proposed that a prolonged stimulus can select for clones of follicular cells with the potential for carcinogenesis. This mechanism may even be involved in the way that feline hyperthyroidism develops over a prolonged period of time. Canine thyroid tumors are rare, but are seen from time to time.

For iodine to do its job, it must be attached to the amino acid tyrosine. Several nutrients are involved in this process including zinc, copper, and vitamins A, B-complex, and C. Good sources of iodine are kelp, Celtic Sea Salt™, fish, sea vegetables, herring, sardines, cod, and shrimp. Good sources of zinc include seafood, oysters, beef, liver, tuna, various cheeses, organ meats, eggs, yeast, dark turkey meat, and various seeds and nuts. The best sources of B-complex vitamins are nutritional yeast, whole grains, and liver.

Once you ensure that your pet has received nutrients to help the thyroid gland, the next step is to make sure that the cells are responding appropriately to the thyroid hormones. This requires the conversion of the less active T_4 to the more active T_3. The trace minerals zinc, copper, and selenium are the required cofactors for iodothyronine iodinase, the enzyme that converts T_4 to the more active T_3. Good sources of selenium are kelp (I use a high selenium-containing kelp), Brazil nuts, saltwater fish, scallops, clams, oysters, wheat germ, brown rice, garlic, sunflower seeds, and green leafy vegetables. Humans living in areas in the world where selenium is deficient have reported a greater incidence of thyroid disease.[33] Selenium deficiency results in low thyroid activity in the cells even though hormone levels are normal or even elevated. The body does not try to correct this problem because the thyroid and pituitary are not affected by a selenium deficiency as much as other cells, so the regulatory feedback system fails. This is a good reason why blood measurement of thyroid hormone levels is not always reliable as to the functional thyroid activity.[34] Most of my canine hypothyroid patients are also put on a high selenium containing kelp, which also contains iodine, zinc, copper, magnesium, sodium, potassium, calcium, chloride, sulfur, iron, and manganese. Remember, hypothyroidism is a serious disease, and unfortunately, the thyroid gland does not regenerate as does the liver. These patients must be supplemented with a name-brand thyroid supplement (I prefer Soloxine). Establishing normal thyroid function is important to optimum health, and minerals in the diet are just as important for good health as thyroid medications. A good natural raw food diet usually provides most of the nutrients needed for prevention of this disease.

Interestingly, the ingestion of iodine is important in the prevention of both hyperthyroidism and hypothyroidism. For example, supplementation of iodine in hyperthyroidism slows or depresses excessive thyroid function, allowing the gland to accept more needed iodine. Supplementation in hypothyroidism allows unsaturated fatty acids to pick up iodine from the thyroid gland, raising blood iodine levels, and improving thyroid function. Iodine appears to have an "adaptogenic" effect on the thyroid gland. It enhances the activity of the thyroid gland in hypothyroidism and slows it down in hyperthyroidism.

chapter 11

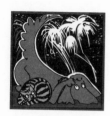

Urinary Tract Diseases and The Protein Diet Controversy

THE CAUSES OF URINARY TRACT DISEASES can range from the bacterial to the psychological (stress) to the unknown. In this chapter, we discuss how holistic as well as traditional methods can offer some relief and cure for patients with urinary tract diseases. We also examine the protein diet controversy: does reduced protein ingestion help patients with renal disease?

CANINE CYSTITIS

By definition, cystitis is inflammation of the urinary bladder. Although the most common cause of canine cystitis is a bacterial infection, that is not necessarily the only cause. Other causes of cystitis may include bladder stones and cancer. A clinical sign of cystitis is frequent urination with or without blood present. Acute infections are easily amenable to antibiotics. Chronic conditions must have a thorough work-up, which includes blood work, urinalysis, cultures, radiographs, and ultrasound. I have found that the use of ultrasonography is the best technique to rule out bladder tumors.

Treatment depends on the cause, and so an accurate diagnosis is imperative. Bladder stones (uroliths) and tumors are best treated with surgical exploration of the bladder. However, if cancer is at the trigone part of the bladder, surgery will not affect a cure; it will only complicate the situation and make things worse. Chronic bacterial infections should be treated with antibiotics and biological response modifiers as well.

History is important in determining a possible cause of cystitis. A common pattern of cystitis patients is that the dog chews and eats plants and grass. Plants and grass tend to produce an alkaline urine (pH 7.4 of higher). The alkaline pH allows bacteria to proliferate and certain crystals to form and irritate and inflame the bladder.

The short-term usage of urinary acidifiers or cranberry juice capsules may help. Reports of the use of cranberry juice for cystitis in humans abound.[1, 2, 3] Interestingly, it is not the acidifying nature of cranberry juice that cures bladder infections. Rather it has been shown that proanthocyanidins are the compounds responsible for preventing the adherence of pathogenic p-fimbriated E. coli to the lining of the urinary tract. According to other investigators, even proanthocyanidins from blueberries show similar activity.[4]

It is important that a natural raw food diet be offered along with clean filtered water. Crystals in the urine may be a function of the difficulty in the digestion of processed dead food. It is unlikely that wolves in the wild develop cystitis.

Though many herbs have been used for urinary tract infections, the most useful herb in most cases of bladder infections is the uva ursi (bearberry). Research has focused on the most important component of bearberry: arbutin. Arbutin is split into glucose and hydroquinone in the kidney, the latter having an antiseptic effect on the urinary tract. However, this only happens if the urine is alkaline.[5] A double-blind study on thirty-seven women with chronic cystitis shows bearberry to be quite effective in the prevention of a recurrence: while the placebo group had a recurrence, no recurrence of the treated group was noted.[6]

Male dogs of the Dalmatian breed tend to produce urate crystals, which eventually form stones in the bladder. This is an obvious genetic fault and must be treated with surgery and an alkalinizing diet. Urinalysis must frequently be performed to evaluate any diet and treatment strategies. More vegetable matter must be added to the diet while offering easily digestible raw meat. Potassium magnesium citrate capsules may also be added to the diet as an alkalinizing agent. Remember, Dalmatians must produce alkaline (pH 7.0 or higher) urine to be free of urate stones, which form in acidic urine (pH 6.0 to 6.5).

FELINE CYSTITIS (FELINE UROLOGICAL SYNDROME)

Feline urological syndrome (FUS) is quite common. Clinical signs include dysuria (painful urination), hematuria (bloody urine), pallakiuria (frequent urination), and urinating in places other than the litter box. History, clinical signs, urinalysis, and radiographs will determine the difference between a diagnosis of FUS or of behavioral disorder. If a male cat's urinary tract is obstructed, the bladder will enlarge with urine and be quite painful when attempting to urinate, with little or no urine expressed. This is an emergency situation and must be handled by a veterinarian immediately, as kidney failure and death will ensue in a short period of time. Female cats, due to a much larger urethra, will not obstruct as the males do.

Unfortunately, with all the research that has gone into this disease, we still call it idiopathic because a specific cause has not been revealed. There are probably multiple causes with diet being at the top of the list. Once again, at least in part, the ingestion of processed, dead, and enzymeless foods plays a major role. It is unlikely that cats in the wild exhibit this disease. This disease is called idiopathic (unknown) because a variety of causes have been postulated, including uroliths (stones), urethral plugs (mucus and debris), bacteria, fungi, parasites, viruses, stress, autoimmune problems, and ingestion of high magnesium and ash-containing foods. Let's look at a few possible causes, keeping in mind that none have been proved as of yet. I would like to see a study with the use of a natural raw food diet (unprocessed) as a preventative in this disease.

One possible cause is the formation of certain types of crystal in the urine. Struvite crystals are the most common crystals, but in one uncontrolled study of 109 cats with FUS, struvite crystals were observed in only 13 percent. The observation that urethral obstruction commonly occurs in cats in the absence of crystalluria (crystals in the urine) indicates that causative factors other than crystaluria may be at work.[7, 8, 9]

Most cats with FUS will be healed in five to seven days whether treated or not. Cats presented at Highlands Veterinary Hospital with this problem have had FUS multiple times in the past, regardless of which "specialized" diet they have tried. These cats have been on antibiotics with a history of it temporarily helping. Interestingly, cats with FUS usually produce a negative urine culture.[10] I have yet to get a positive urine culture with this disease in cats, unlike in dogs, where urine culture is always positive. Of course, there is a possibility that the reason for a negative urine culture is that there may be uncommon or rare or even difficult to culture bacteria. This seems not to be the case, since this has already been postulated with futile results.[11] If bacteria are not the cause, then antibiotics are not the answer. Anecdotal reports by pet owners or veterinarians that antibiotics help is probably coincidental. Remember, most cases will resolve with or without treatment in five to seven days.

Viruses of various types have been implicated, incriminated, and isolated, but not proven as of yet in this disease.[12] They may be normal inhabitants within bladder cells or pathogenic when the immune system is compromised or suppressed.

Some researchers compared FUS in cats with interstitial cystitis in humans.[13] An autoimmune or immune-mediated inflammation has been implicated in interstitial cystitis in humans, and although it has not been proven in FUS, I believe there is reason to find that an autoimmune component has strong possibilities. Perhaps at certain times there are toxic components in the urine that irritate the bladder wall. At times, a cat may have indiscriminate eating habits, particularly outdoor cats eating plants or grass. However, I also see this in strictly indoor cats that do not eat plants. This may add to the inflammatory process in FUS.

Acute or chronic stressful situations can suppress the immune system and predispose us and our pets to a host of diseases. During stress, many complicated hormonal and immunological changes occur. Although some stress may be beneficial, the adaptive responses to stress may themselves become stressors capable of inducing disease. Almost any stressful situation such as earthquakes, moving, weather changes, and diet changes has been implicated in recurrent episodes of FUS in cats.[14] One of my patients exhibits signs of cystitis whenever relatives from out of town visit and stay for a few days. Its cystitis quickly resolves when the relatives leave. There are certainly other causes implicated in this disease; however, none have been proved and more research is needed in its prevention.

Many of my chronic cystitis patients respond to biological response modifiers and a natural raw food diet. Remember, food is much easier to digest when it is alive with nutrients and enzymes. Perhaps dead processed food aggravates the situation by causing an inflammatory process during digestion. Perhaps our pets' wild feline relatives have the answers to our questions.

KIDNEY DISEASE

The kidneys are two bean-shaped organs located below the rib cage in the mid-back area. They are responsible for ridding the body of waste material and controlling the volume and composition of body fluids.

Within each kidney are about a million units called nephrons.

These nephrons consist of filtering units called glomeruli, which are attached to tubules. When blood enters each glomeruli, it is filtered and the remaining fluid passes along the tubule, where water and chemicals are either removed from or added to the filtered fluid, depending on what the body needs. The final product is the urine, which is eliminated via the bladder. Specific kidney functions include:

1. Regulation of water and electrolyte balances, by filtering and reabsorbing potassium, magnesium, chloride, sodium, etc.

2. Maintenance of blood pressure by maintaining adequate water volume, filtering and reabsorbing sodium, and synthesizing renin, kinin, and prostaglandins (steroids and nonsteroidal anti-inflammatory drugs inhibit prostaglandins).

3. Filtration and excretion of metabolic waste products such as blood urea nitrogen (BUN), urea, uric acid, and creatinine. BUN and creatinine are also secreted.

4. Filtration and excretion of foreign chemicals (drugs, toxins, synthetic vitamins).

5. Secretion of hormones such as erythropoietin (which acts on the stem cells of the bone marrow to stimulate red blood cell production, 90 percent of which is made in the kidneys and 10 percent in the liver), renin, kinins, and prostaglandins.

6. Involvement with gluconeogenesis (the kidneys form glucose from amino acids and other precursors during prolonged fasting).

7. Regulation of acid-based balance by bicarbonate reabsorption and hydrogen in secretions, maintenance of calcium and phosphorus balance, hydroxylation of vitamin D to 1-25 dihydroxycholecalciferol, and filtration and reabsorption of phosphate and calcium (dependent on PTH).

8. Maintenance of hematocrit/hemoglobin by synthesis of erythropoietin.

About 21 percent of the cardiac output flows to the kidneys. Each kidney has about one million nephrons (the functional unit of the kidney). The nephron consists of two parts: the glomerulus, where fluid and some solutes are filtered from the blood, and the tubule, which converts the fluid into urine through reabsorption of solutes and fluid, as well as secreting solutes and fluid into the tubules via the peritubular capillaries. Most plasma substances pass freely into the glomerular filtrate with the exception of proteins. Once in the tubule, water and specific solutes are reabsorbed as well as secreted via the peritubular capillaries. Waste products such as urea, creatinine, uric acid, and urates are poorly reabsorbed. Some waste products such as creatine and BUN are additionally secreted from the blood into the tubules. Electrolytes such as sodium ions, chloride ions, and bicarbonate ions are highly reabsorbed, so little appear in the urine. Nutritional substances such as amino acids and glucose are completely reabsorbed. In diabetic animals, they will appear in the urine.

The kidney cannot regenerate new nephrons. Renal injury, disease, and aging will decrease the number of nephrons. It is estimated in humans that after age forty the functional nephrons begin to decrease by 10 percent each year due to benign nephrosclerosis. The remaining nephrons adapt to take on the increased workload. Up to 75 percent of the functional nephrons can be lost before clinical symptoms appear. This is one reason veterinarians recommend a geriatric work-up yearly for both dogs and cats past the age of ten. With kidney failure, death is due to a combination of acidosis, a high concentration of potassium, toxins, and accumulation of fluid. The kidneys are no longer able to produce urine.

In cases such as urethral obstruction in male cats or infectious nephritis, it is imperative to institute aggressive fluid therapy as well as to relieve obstruction as soon as possible to prevent chronic renal failure. Preventing chronic kidney failure is a better goal than treating chronic kidney failure.

Monitoring of kidney function is easily accomplished by blood testing and urinalysis. Parameters used are blood urea nitrogen (BUN), creatinine, phosphorus, cholesterol, and urine specific gravity (urine concentration).

Clinical signs of kidney disease include increased drinking and urination, dehydration, anorexia, vomiting, weight loss, anemia, lethargy, dry skin, and an "unthrifty appearance."

To understand how the various herbs benefit the kidneys, it is important to understand how the kidneys function at the cellular level. There is a rationale behind the usage of various herbal therapeutics. Platelet activating factor (PAF) is an inflammatory mediator that plays an important role in allergic and inflammatory processes, including ischemic renal failure. Evidence for involvement of PAF in renal immune injury (glomerulonephritis) has been provided by the observation that PAF is released during kidney allograft rejection (kidney transplant). It has been proposed that PAF participates in glomerular immune complex deposition in experimental serum sickness and also in systemic lupus erythematosis. Research shows it is released by isolated perfused kidneys and glomeruli as well as by suspensions of medullary cells, although not by tubules. The mesangial cells are thought to be the major source of PAF in the glomerulus. Mesangial cells located between epithelial cells are believed to provide structural support to the glomerular basement membrane. In addition, these cells are part of a defensive system and have phagocytic properties. Inflammatory conditions will produce mesangial cell hyperplasia and increase the phagocytic function in these cells.[15] PAF has been shown to cause renal vasoconstriction and release of inflammatory agents such as prostaglandins and thromboxane B_2 in the kidney. There are specific binding sites for PAF. PAF antagonists interfere with the binding of PAF to its cellular receptors. In short, this causes kidney damage.

Interestingly, ginkgolides from ginkgo biloba are naturally occurring platelet-activating factor antagonists. Ginkgo is a versatile herb that I have used in many degenerative diseases. Ginkgolides inhibit PAF-induced release of thromboxane B_2 and prostaglandins from primary cultures of human and rat glomerular mesangial cells. Ginkgo also inhibits PAF-induced formation of reactive oxygen species from cultured mesangial cells and destruction of the glomeruli (ginkgo is known to be an antioxidant, which is important since free radical production is implicated in progressive kidney disorders). In addition, this antagonist inhibits PAF-induced decreases in renal blood flow, glomerular filtration, and urinary sodium excretion.[16] Caution should be exercised when giving ginkgo to dogs that are taking aspirin, as this may prolong bleeding times. One study using a ginkgo extract (BN52021) showed that it reduced proteinuria and histopathological lesions in nephrotoxic rabbits. Additionally, this extract given intravenously prior to renal graft surgery and for four days after surgery has been shown to increase the chance of graft survival and decrease the number of acute rejection episodes after surgery.[17]

ACUTE RENAL FAILURE (ARF)
There are several mechanisms that will predispose a pet to acute renal failure.

Prerenal (ARF)
Prerenal acute renal failure is associated with reduced cardiac

output and low blood pressure, or conditions associated with diminished blood volume and low blood pressure, such as severe hemorrhage and shock. As long as renal blood flow does not fall below 20 percent of normal, acute renal failure can usually be reversed if the cause is corrected before renal cell damage occurs. When the blood flow to the kidneys decreases, the glomerular filtration rate (GFR) also decreases. This decreases the kidneys' workload, and therefore decreases the kidneys' requirement for energy and oxygen. Ischemia (decreased oxygen) cannot persist for more than a few hours at below 20 percent blood flow, or the kidneys will experience intrarenal acute renal failure.

Nephrotoxic (ARF)

Nephrotoxic or intrarenal acute renal failure is due to abnormalities of the kidney itself, including those affecting the blood vessels, glomeruli, or tubules. Tubular necroses are many and varied and include ethylene glycol poisoning, heavy metals, aminoglycosides, cis-platinum, carbo-platinum, nonsteroidal anti-inflammatory drugs, snake venom, hypercalcemia, angiotensin-converting-enzyme inhibitors, pyelonephritis, diabetes mellitus, and glomerulonephritis.

Postrenal (ARF)

Postrenal acute renal failure is commonly seen in urethral obstruction in male cats. However, this also is occasionally seen in urethral obstruction in male dogs as well.

Treatment of acute renal failure requires prompt hospitalization and aggressive IV fluid therapy, correction of electrolyte imbalance, and identifying the cause. This is an immediate life-threatening situation, and time is of the essence. Antioxidants, along with herbs that are used in chronic kidney failure, are good adjuncts to intravenous fluid therapy.

Chronic Renal Failure

Chronic renal failure is due to irreversible loss of large numbers of functioning nephrons. Clinical symptoms occur when there are fewer than 30 percent normal functioning nephrons. In general, chronic renal failure occurs due to the same reasons acute renal failure occurs, but the progression is slower. Often the initial insult to the kidney leads to progressive deterioration of kidney function and increased loss of nephrons over time until the patient reaches end-stage renal failure. When nephrons are lost, other nephrons take on a larger load. They adapt and excrete normal amounts of water and solutes, until the kidney is reduced by 20 to 30 percent of the normal nephron mass. Over the years, the glomeruli are injured. It is thought this injury is caused by the increased pressure and stretch from the increased blood pressure on the glomeruli. This eventually causes scar tissue and further destruction of the kidneys. The only method known by conventional medicine to slow the glomerular damage down is to lower blood pressure and glomerular hydrostatic pressure by using drugs such as angiotensin-converting enzyme inhibitors to block formation of angiotension II (Vasotec/Enalapril). This drug increases sodium and water excretion while producing vasodilatation in glomeruli. Chronic renal failure is insidious and is usually seen in older pets, particularly older cats. Most practices such as Highlands Veterinary Hospital see far more feline patients than canine patients with chronic renal failure.

The most important tool you have for prevention of renal failure is recognition of the leading causes of renal failure. Most patients are usually over ten years of age. You can prevent or slow down renal failure only if you treat it in the early stages. Clinical symptoms show up when there is 70 percent destruction of functional nephrons. Laboratory profiles of kidney failure show up much sooner. Abnormal blood cholesterol, BUN, creatinine, and phosphorus may be seen in all or some profiles. In the feline patient, elevated cholesterol may be a better indicator of kidney disease than BUN. I have seen cats with moderate BUN levels but high cholesterol levels die of chronic kidney failure. Hypercholesterolemia in cats is a definite causative factor for additional kidney damage.

Before discussing various herbal treatment options and the protein diet controversy, I must emphasize that the administration of daily subcutaneous fluids at home is probably the most important treatment option. Most cats will receive about 200 cc's of lactated ringers solution on a daily or every-other-day basis depending on clinical signs and laboratory indices.

HERBAL TREATMENT OPTIONS

Astragalus Membranaceus
Astragalus acts as a diuretic when the kidneys are weak. It provides support for the kidneys and has been used in Chinese medicine for treatment for chronic kidney disease. Astragalus is thought to increase renal blood flow. It is anti-inflammatory, hepatoprotective, an immune enhancer, and an antioxidant. It helps restore normal tissue tone and function.

Chitosan
Chitosan is a natural derivative of "chitin," which is found in the exoskeletons of crabs, shrimp, and other shellfish. Chitosan attracts fat by actually binding negatively charged fatty acids to its positively charged fiber. Chitosan forms a bond with fat, which cannot be absorbed by the body; instead, it is passed through to the colon and out of the body. In addition, as the bonded complex of fat and chitosan moves into the small intestine, it also binds with bile acids and cholesterol. The importance if chitosan is that it lowers blood urea nitrogen (BUN), creatinine, and cholesterol.[18]

Cordyceps
Cordyceps is one of my favorite and most versatile herbs. The view of traditional Chinese medicine is that cordyceps supports the normal function and strengthens the energy of the kidneys and nourishes the body's chi or vital force. In fact, research with cordyceps has shown that it produces definite beneficial effects on the kidneys.[19] Cordyceps has been found to cause a profound

promotion of DNA synthesis in kidney cells, which indicates enhanced regeneration of damaged cells.[20]

The effect of cordyceps on the kidney was tested in a double-blind, placebo-controlled trial in fifty-two patients at a hospital in Nanjing, China. The patient volunteers had not suffered from kidney disease in the past, and their kidney function was normal. After random division of the patients into two groups, one group received cordyceps and the other received a placebo. Both groups, composed of men and women, received injections of aminoglycoside antibiotics (toxin), which interfere with normal functions of the kidneys. Results showed that those on the placebo developed greatly elevated signs of kidney toxicity, but the group on cordyceps was protected.[21]

Another study in China reported that cordyceps can help patients with chronic renal failure. A clinical study of thirty-seven chronic renal failure patients treated with a daily dosage of five grams of cordyceps for thirty days found significant improvements. Compared with the results of pre-treatment tests, red blood cells and hemoglobin counts were greatly increased. The most improvement was shown in a creatinine clearance test, which measures the kidney filtration rate in terms of a waste product called serum creatinine. Tests showed an improvement rate of about 39 percent. In addition, there was a 34 percent decrease in blood urea nitrogen (BUN). A high level of BUN is a major indicator of kidney disease, heart failure, dehydration, intestinal bleeding, muscle degeneration, and an increased breakdown of protein. The test subjects also showed increased levels of superoxide dismutase (SOD), one of the body's free radical scavengers. The arterial blood pressure of test subjects dropped by an average of 15 percent. Equally important was the 63 percent drop in proteins found in their urine, which is one of the strongest indicators of an overall correction of kidney function.[22]

A high level of a protein known as epidermal growth factor (EGF) also was found in the urine of patients taking cordyceps. This led researchers to suggest the increase in EGF may be involved in the role of kidney protection by cordyceps. Research with EGF in kidney disease is of considerable interest. Various research groups have found that, in acute kidney failure in animals, the administration of EGF increased the rate of recovery.[23]

Enzyme Therapy

I prefer to use super oxide desmutase (SOD) and wobenzyme, an enteric coated pancreatic enzyme tablet. SOD is a potent antioxidant that helps to minimize free radical damage and enhances the body's antioxidant capability.

It is important to note that systemic enzyme therapy is not necessarily used to aid digestion, but to reduce pain, swelling, and inflammation in the kidneys and to stimulate the immune system, helping to reduce circulating antigen-antibody complexes. Enzymes improve circulation, help speed tissue repair, bring nutrients to the damaged area, remove waste products, improve health, strengthen the body as a whole, and build general resistance.

Essential Fatty Acids

Omega-3 fatty acids have been shown to help patients with kidney failure. Good sources are flax oil, crushed flax seeds, raw meat, raw milk, fish, sardines, and seafood. Many popular processed kidney diets claim to have omega-3 fatty acids. The problem with these diets is that omega-3 fatty acids are easily destroyed and oxidized in the processing of these foods. The ingestion of rancid fatty acids could cause free radical damage—in other words, they could cause more harm than good. These foods are misleading, and there is nothing about these foods that is beneficial to the kidneys.

Panax Ginseng

Oral ginseng has been shown to decrease uremic toxins such as creatinine, methylguanidine, and guanidinosuccinic acid. One study in rats found oral ginseng demonstrated the arrest of progressive renal disorder; it suppressed uremic toxins, decreased urinary excretion of proteins, and inhibited mesangial proliferation. In experiments using cultured mesangial cells, there was considerable suppression of mesangial proliferation. This suggests ginseng has a role as a free radical scavenger. Ginseng's action as a free radical scavenger is important since free radical production is implicated in progressive kidney disorders.[24]

Recancostat (Stabilized Glutathione)
This is a combination of stabilized glutathione and anthocyanins. Glutathione is one of the most important antioxidants in the body. It helps slow down the degenerative processes. Remember, raw eggs and raw milk are great sources of precursors to glutathione.

Rehmannia
This herb increases blood flow to the kidneys and helps ward off urinary infections as well. I prefer to use a combination called Rehmannia Eight, which contains rehmannia, cornus, dioscorea, hoelen, alisma, aconite, cinnamon, and moutan. According to traditional Chinese medicine, this combination increases kidney chi. Rehmannia contains potent polysaccharides that support the functions of the kidney and bladder.[25]

Rheum Officinalis (Rhubarb)
Rhubarb increases glomerular filtration and decreases cholesterol and triglyceride levels. Interactions of lipids with advanced glycosylation have been implicated in human diabetic patients with kidney disease. Rheum has been shown to relieve diabetic nephropathy in humans by improving lipid metabolism. An extract of rhubarb has been shown to increase urinary excretion of urea nitrogen and creatinine, probably due to increased glomerular filtration.[26] Rhubarb is also quite helpful in constipation. I use this herb on an as-needed basis to avoid "lazy colon," which can develop from rhubarb's colon-stimulating effects. This herb increases circulation, especially in the kidneys and gastrointestinal tract, while decreasing hypertension.

Renatrophin PMG
This is a glandular product made from bovine kidneys. Produced by Standard Process Labs, renatrophin PMG has all the nutrients designed by nature for healthy kidneys. Remember, cats are particularly sensitive to natural taurine, which is destroyed when meat is cooked. Interestingly, big cats in captivity can live well into their twenties, while in the wild they may only live twelve to fifteen years. In captivity, they are fed raw meat as would be eaten in the wild, except that now stress is minimized or absent. Raw meat is crucial for a cat's diet.

Salvia Miltiorrhiza
Salvia miltiorrhiza is a traditional Chinese medicinal herb used in human treatment of such afflictions as hemorrhage, menstrual disorders, swelling, and coronary heart disease. Salvia's active ingredients include diterpenoids, polyphenolic acids, and a flavanone. The crude extract and polyphenolic acid have been found to improve renal function in vitro (test tube) and in vivo (live animal).[27]

One important constituent, known as magnesium lithospermate B, has been shown to decrease blood urea nitrogen, serum creatinine, methylguanidine (oxidative product), guanidinosuccinic acid (oxidative product), and inorganic phosphate in uremic rats whose uremic state had been induced by an adenine diet. It works by activating the kallikrein-kinin system in the rat kidney to promote the production and secretion of prostaglandin E2 (PGE2), inducing dilation of renal blood vessels, and increasing the renal blood flow and glomerular filtration rate. PGE2 also inhibits proliferation of mesangial cells and acts antagonistically against vasoconstriction brought about from thromboxane A2. PGE2 has been found to inhibit tubular reabsorption of sodium, thus lowering hypertension.[28, 29]

Vinpocetine
Vinpocetine is a derivative of vincamine, which is an extract of

the periwinkle plant. Vinpocetine is often used for treatment of cerebral circulatory disorders such as memory problems, acute stroke, motor disorders, dizziness, and other cerebro-vestibular (inner ear) problems. However, it has also been shown to increase myocardial and renal capillary perfusion.[30] This is a safe herb that I have used in both dogs and cats with good success.

THE PROTEIN DIET CONTROVERSY

This is a controversial subject in both human and veterinary medicine, as there is little or no scientific basis for precise recommendations for reduced protein ingestion by patients with reduced renal function. Dietary protein restriction has been widely accepted as a form of nutritional management for animals with reduced renal function for more than fifty years. This is based on a study done on rats predisposed to renal failure.[31] There are many misconceptions and myths surrounding this subject matter.

I personally have never seen a patient increase its life span or quality of life with a restricted protein diet. To the contrary, patients fed a higher or normal protein diet tend to have enhanced feelings of well-being. Higher protein diets tend to be more palatable as well.

There are many *false assumptions* pointing to reduced protein intake in regard to renal disease that have been perpetuated by food companies for many years. They include:

1. Decreased protein intake increases life expectancy.

2. Decreased protein intake increases quality of life.

3. High dietary protein intake injures kidneys.

4. Reduced protein intake slows the progression of renal disease.

5. Protein intake results in uremic toxins.

6. Increased urea causes increased workload for the kidneys.

It should be remembered that fifty or sixty years ago when these myths were perpetuated not much was known about the kidneys. For example, in 1947 it was reported that blood urea concentration was an accurate measure of kidney function and the concept of extrarenal azotemia (excess amounts of nitrogen in blood) was first reported.[32] It was then believed that moderate protein restriction was beneficial to human patients. This fallacy fell out of favor when it was realized that kidney workload is closely tied to active sodium reabsorption and that urea was passively handled. Therefore, dietary restrictions were not thought to be needed in human patients with chronic renal failure because of the lack of evidence that a normal protein intake had a deleterious effect on the kidneys.

Unfortunately, even the National Research Council (NRC) of the National Academy of Sciences adapted this theory in 1972.[33] The council was also duped by antiquated science. It accepted the theory that high protein found in some commercial diets increases the workload of the liver and kidney and contributes to renal disease in dogs. There is absolutely no evidence to support this view, and the recommendation has since been dropped. There is, however, overwhelming evidence that high protein diets enhance renal function in normal dogs. This has led to confusion among veterinarians and food manufacturers who have been told for decades that low protein diets may be beneficial for kidney function and therefore high protein diets may be deleterious to normal dogs.

There are many experimental studies on dogs that have failed to provide evidence of the benefit of reduced dietary protein to influence the course of renal failure.[34-39] Modern research has clearly shown that the concept of increased workload, protein intake causing injury to the kidneys, and reduced protein intake slowing the progression of renal disease are incorrect.

Some may argue that the benefits of reduced protein intake in animals with chronic renal failure (CRF) include decreased serum urea nitrogen and phosphorus concentrations. However, there are undesirable effects associated with restricting dietary protein in dogs and cats with CRF. If dietary protein is restricted in relation to the animal's protein needs, reduced glomerular filtration rate (GFR), protein depletion (decreased body weight, muscle mass, and serum albumin concentration), anemia, and acidosis will occur or be aggravated. Just as increased dietary protein results in increased glomerular filtration, restricted dietary protein is associated with a reduction in GFR. Exacerbation of the anemia of chronic renal failure occurs because protein depletion further compromises erythrogenesis (red blood cell production).

When feeding protein-reduced diets, it must be kept in mind that the energy requirements of the body have a higher priority than does protein anabolism; therefore, if the available carbohydrates and fats are insufficient to meet calorie requirements, endogenous (from body) proteins are often broken down as a source of energy. Catabolism (breaking down) of endogenous proteins for energy increases the nitrogenous waste the kidney must excrete and exacerbates the clinical signs of renal failure. It is imperative to realize that minimum protein requirements for dogs and cats with chronic renal failure are actually higher than those of normal dogs and cats. In other words, there are disadvantages to restricted protein diets. These include reduced kidney function as measured by GFR and renal plasma flow, a negative nitrogen balance, and the aggravation of a catabolic state in the presence of proteinuria.

Pets with CRF must be on a raw food and raw meat diet. Raw meat is bland, and some pets must become accustomed to it over time. If palatability is a problem, try mixing raw meat with palatable canned or baby food. These pets deserve to eat anything they find palatable. Raw eggs with a higher omega-3 content, along with raw milk, are excellent choices as well. (See chapter 2 on nutrition and chapter 5 on raw meat diets.)

chapter 12

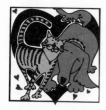

Herbs With Cardiovascular Effects

CONGESTIVE HEART FAILURE OCCURS WHEN THE HEART IS UNABLE TO PUMP BLOOD THROUGHOUT THE BODY (but not all patients with heart failure have congestion). There are two categories of congestive heart failure: systolic and diastolic. In the systolic type of the disease, blood coming into the heart from the lungs may be regurgitated so that fluid accumulates in the lungs (pulmonary congestion). In the diastolic type, the heart muscle becomes stiff and cannot relax, leading to an accumulation of fluid in the legs and abdomen.

Congestive heart failure is in itself not a diagnosis. Rather it is the physiological result of damage to the heart caused by some underlying condition. Therefore, it is not enough to say that an animal has congestive heart failure. The congestive heart failure (CHF) has to be due to some underlying process, and successful treatment is dependent upon that recognition. Many veterinarians and physicians consider the cause of most heart problems as idiopathic (unknown); however, I believe that the majority are due to malnutrition. Certainly, there are the genetic exceptions such as cardiomyopathy in Doberman pinschers, but the vast majority are due to nutritional insufficiency, as we will see later.

Cardiomyopathy is a condition in which the heart muscle is damaged and no longer functions properly. It is divided into three categories: dilated, hypertrophic, and restricted. Dilated cardiomyopathy, where the heart muscle becomes thin and stretched, may be caused by unknown factors (idiopathic), malnutrition, endocrine factors, or genetic factors. Restrictive cardiomyopathy results when some disease process restricts the movement of the heart. Hypertrophic cardiomyopathy, where the heart muscle becomes enlarged and thickened, is due to high blood pressure and failure of the heart's valves.

A number of generalized symptoms are associated with heart failure. They include lethargy, fluid accumulation (edema), coughing, and respiratory distress. Heart failure generally develops slowly, and the pet owner is often unaware of the condition until symptoms appear.

In most cases, the diagnosis of heart disease is made after the veterinarian has conducted a physical exam, radiographs, ECG, and echocardiogram. A blood panel should always be performed to rule out any metabolic or hormonal problems.

Although congestive heart failure can be treated and improved by therapy, it is important to treat the underlying cause to prevent progression and worsening of symptoms leading to death.

CONVENTIONAL TREATMENTS OF HEART DISEASE

Various types of medications are used in the treatment of CHF, each of which has a different function. ACE (angiotensin-converting enzyme) inhibitors and vasodilators expand blood vessels, thereby allowing the heart to function more efficiently. Beta-blockers reduce oxygen demand in the left ventricle, which is often damaged in patients with CHF. Digitalis increases the pumping action of the heart, and diuretics eliminate fluid accumulation. In many cases, successful control of hypertension can alleviate symptoms. ACE inhibitors and diuretics are the most popular drugs used in veterinary medicine. I have used a combination of Western drugs, nutrition, and herbs to successfully treat many seriously ill CHF patients.

Diuretics lower blood pressure by reducing the volume of fluid in blood and body tissues; they promote the elimination of salt and water through increased urination. Diuretics work by reducing the fluid volume being forced through the arteries, and by relaxing the smaller arteries of the body, allowing them to expand and increase the total fluid capacity of the arterial system. The net result of diuretics is lower pressure due to reduced volume in an expanded arterial space.

ACE inhibitors prevent the formation of active angiotensin, a substance that increases both the fluid volume and degree of constriction of the blood vessels. By inhibiting the formation of this compound, ACE inhibitors relax the arterial walls and reduce fluid volume. Do not think that all drugs are bad; in fact, ACE inhibitors actually improve heart function and increase blood and oxygen flow to the heart, liver, and kidneys. The actions of ACE inhibitors indicate that these drugs actually reduce mortality and increase quality of life. ACE inhibitors are generally well tolerated; however, there have been reports of kidney damage in some patients. Caution should be exercised when using diuretics and ACE inhibitors together. Blood tests should be monitored on a regular basis because ACE inhibitors can cause the body to retain potassium, which can exacerbate heart and kidney problems.

TAKING A NUTRITIONAL APPROACH TO CHF

From a nutritional aspect, heart muscle cells are composed of eighteen different amino acids, all of which must be supplied simultaneously and unaltered. Six of the eighteen are heat labile; so when food is cooked, pasteurized, or otherwise heated, these six amino acids are denatured and then coagulated to an insoluble state which the body cannot use to form polypeptide chains needed for cellular repair or replacement. About ten years ago, it was noted that some cats acquired cardiomyopathy due to the destruction of taurine in processed or cooked protein sources. These so-called 100 percent balanced diets had to be supplemented with taurine. Taurine in its isolated state does not have the same effect on the body as when in its natural synergistic undenatured raw state. Cats are particularly sensitive to the need of this amino acid, especially in its natural state. Unfortunately, the addition of taurine in the diet has not totally eliminated cardiomyopathy in cats. I must emphasize again that excellent sources of all amino acids in their natural synergistic state are raw meat, raw eggs, raw milk, and raw fish. Cats must not be fed a strictly fish diet as this may cause steitis or inflammation of their fat, and eventual death. It is important to always vary the diets of both dogs and cats. (We'll discuss taurine's relation to other nutrients in additional detail later in this chapter.)

Cardiac muscle cells are also rich in myoglobin (an oxygen carrier) as well as enzymes involved in the electron transport chain and the Krebs citric acid cycle (series of reactions involving oxidative metabolism of pyruvic acid and liberation of energy). From the electron transport chain and citric acid cycle, heart muscle cells obtain energy for contraction by the biochemical conversion process called ATP. This energy system, which converts fuel (food) into cellular energy, is located in the mitochondria of the cells and is oxidative phosphorylation. Interestingly, beef heart mitochondria was found to contain a structure called electron transport particle (ETP), which contains the entire electron transport chain from nicotinamide adenine dinacleotide (NAD) to oxygen. ETP contains two hemes (iron-containing blood pigment): one red and one green. The green heme contains tyrosinase (enzyme combined with organic copper). ETP also contains a flavin (B_2), a copper flavin, and a lipid, which apparently is a source of vitamin K and coenzyme Q_{10} (CoQ_{10}).[1] Vitamin C complex plays an obvious, important role here. Since beef heart mitochondria contain the complete electron transport particle plus the cofactors of the citric and fatty acid cycles, then if the proteins of the beef heart cells have not been destroyed by heat processing, ingestion of raw beef heart could greatly benefit heart failure patients.

Coenzyme Q_{10}

Coenzyme Q_{10} has become quite popular in the supplementation of heart patients. There are at least seventeen reactions in the body to yield CoQ_{10} from the amino acid phenylalanine and acetyl CoA. Many nutrients are required for the production of CoQ_{10}. We do not know yet the whole story, but some of the nutrients involved are B_2, B_3, B_5, B_6, B_{12}, vitamin C complex, and others. Chemically, CoQ_{10} is similar to vitamin K, and is found in the chloroplasts of green plants as well as beef heart cells. The chloroplasts provide a chlorophyll/vitamin E complex, which is involved in the electron transport system. What is important is that this type of vitamin E is rich in selenium, the trace mineral activator of vitamin E complex and an important factor needed for the synthesis of CoQ_{10} in the body. Within the electron transport particle (ETP) of beef heart cells is found a fat source of CoQ_{10}. CoQ_{10} is essential to ETP and when coupled to oxidative phosphorylation is needed for heart muscle tone and contractile strength. Since the normal heart is higher in coenzyme Q_{10} content than most other tissues, it follows that when samples are taken from heart disease patients, a deficiency of coenzyme Q_{10} is observed.[2]

Coenzyme Q_{10} functions as a fat-soluble vitamin and is found in every cell of the body. Since it is synthesized by cells from required raw materials, it would not be categorized as a vitamin according to classical definitions (vitamins can be acquired only through food). Classification is not important; however, I suspect that just as elderly humans that have been found to be deficient in coenzyme Q_{10}, elderly pets too are probably low or deficient in CoQ_{10} as well.

CoQ_{10} is an essential component in a fundamental biochemical process, namely the conversion of fuel into cellular energy (ATP). The highest concentrations appear in the heart and liver, so beef heart and liver are excellent food sources. CoQ_{10} is found in other foods such as beans, eggs, fish (especially codfish, mackerel, salmon, and sardines), fish oil, spinach, whole grains (especially the germ), vegetable oils, and organ meats. Coincidentally, these foods are also good sources of vitamin E complex, which synergistically enhances CoQ_{10}'s effects.[3]

We have already seen how selenium has a close relationship with vitamin E and, in fact, may be its activating element. Selenium appears to also have an important relationship with CoQ_{10}. It is known that levels of CoQ_{10} decline in selenium deficiency and that selenium stimulates CoQ_{10} production. Therefore, adequate selenium is required to produce the necessary coenzyme Q_{10} required for a healthy heart. As can be seen, selenium, vitamin E complex, and coenzyme Q_{10} have an intimate relationship in the maintenance of a healthy heart, but they are certainly not the only nutrients that a healthy heart requires.

Numerous studies have demonstrated the value and effectiveness of CoQ_{10} supplementation.[4-10] In studies on congestive heart failure, human patients given CoQ_{10} supplementation often improved dramatically, resuming normal activities. Other cardiovascular areas, the immune system, diabetes, other muscle tissues, nervous tissues, the retina, periodontal tissues, and general energy have all benefited from coenzyme Q_{10} supplementation.

Unfortunately, CoQ_{10} supplementation is expensive due to a Japanese monopoly; CoQ_{10} supplement is manufactured in Japan. It is important to remember that supplements of coenzyme Q_{10} are synthesized as pure refined manufactured compound by fermentation. I recommend and use the oil-soluble capsules, as they have been shown to be three times as effective as the powdered capsule form. In reality, this is actually more of a drug than a food and is certainly no substitute for a raw food diet. CoQ_{10} is a supplement to a good diet, not a substitute.

For pets with heart disease, I prescribe coenzyme Q_{10} along with various herbs and an important supplement from Standard Process Labs called Cardio-Plus. Cardio-Plus is an all-natural food concentrate composed of bovine heart protomorphogen

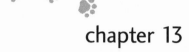

chapter 13

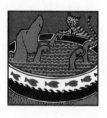

Natural Approaches to Respiratory Diseases

ASTHMA

THE WORD ASTHMA IS DERIVED FROM THE GREEK LANGUAGE AND MEANS "DIFFICULT BREATHING." In this chapter, we will be discussing bronchial asthma, in which a narrowing of the airways occurs due to contraction, or spasm, of smooth muscle, edema (swelling) of the bronchial mucosa, and increased mucus within the bronchial lumen (canal). In other words, bronchial asthma can be defined as airway obstruction, inflammation, and a hyperresponsiveness to various stimuli. It is estimated that more than half of all humans living with asthma have chronic inflammation with:

1. Increased collagen production and deposition beneath the basement membrane.

2. Disruption of the epithelial tissue.

3. Increased numbers of both mast cells and eosinophils (two major components of inflammation).

HOW THE INFLAMMATORY PROCESS OCCURS IN ASTHMA

Let's review the inflammatory process since it is a key mechanism in explaining the pathologic changes seen in asthma. Inflammation of the airways causes the epithelial lining to be damaged. This gives noxious stimuli access to the underlying smooth muscle, submucosal mast cells, and the cholinergic irritant receptors found in the junction between the cells. To understand the natural approaches to asthma, it is important to understand the major players in the disorder: the inflammatory cells, the mediators, the role of mucus production, airway smooth muscle, and nervous system.

The Inflammatory Cells

1. **Mast Cells.** Mast cells are found throughout the walls of the respiratory tract and are believed to be important in the immediate response to allergens. When the allergen is bound to IgE, the mast cells set off an alarm by releasing many inflammatory mediators such as histamine, eosinophils, neutrophil chemotactic factor, prostaglandin, and platelet activating factor (PAF). It has been reported that serotonin is a primary mediator in feline mast cells.[1] This mediator is absent in dogs, horses, and human airways. During an acute asthmatic attack, inhaled antigens within the airways cause acute mast cell degranulation and release of preformed serotonin; this then causes the sudden contraction of airway smooth muscle. Furthermore, it has long been assumed that histamine released from feline mast cells caused acute bronchoconstriction. This assumption is probably incorrect. In fact, histamine may actually dilate feline airways through

an H_3 receptor found in the airway smooth muscle of cats, but not in humans, dogs, or horses.

2. **Eosinophils.** Eosinophils contain basic protein, which appears to be responsible for much of the damage to the epithelial tissue lining the airway. Eosinophils have been found in high numbers in the mucus of asthmatic patients.

3. **Lung macrophages.** The macrophages found in the lung are responsible for clearing away bacteria and other "foreign" debris. When a macrophage encounters a substance that must be removed, it releases inflammatory mediators such as platelet activating factor (PAF) and leukotrienes. Macrophages also release eosinophils and neutrophil chemotactic factor, which puts out a call to these cells to come assist in the work.

The Inflammatory Mediators

1. **Prostaglandin.** When arachidonic acid is released from the cell membrane, it can be broken down by the enzyme cyclooxygenase to form prostaglandin. Various prostaglandins appear to have a role in inflammation and bronchoconstriction, which occurs in asthma.

2. **Leukotrienes.** Arachidonic acid can also be broken down through another pathway involving the enzyme lipooxygenase to produce leukotrienes. Leukotrienes make up the slow-reacting substances of anaphylaxis. When these substances are released, they decrease mucociliary clearance as well as increase microvascular permeability leading to increased airway edema and bronchoconstriction.

3. **Thromboxanes.** Thromboxane A_2 is released by a number of cells including lung macrophages, fibroblasts, neutrophils, and lung platelets. This substance plays a role in the

bronchoconstriction, which occurs in the late asthmatic response and also appears to be involved in the hyperreactivity and inflammation that develop.

4. **Platelet activating factor.** Platelet activating factor (PAF) is produced by a number of cells in the lung including macrophages, eosinophils, and neutrophils. PAF causes the immediate bronchoconstriction seen in asthma, and is the only substance known to sustain increased bronchial hyperreactivity.

Role of Mucus

Mucus is composed of approximately 5 percent glycoproteins and 95 percent water, and is produced by the epithelial and goblet cells located in the bronchioles. The lumen of the airways is continually lined by a thin layer of mucus, which is controlled by active ion transport across the epithelium. Ions move across the epithelium, and water moves into the lumen. Mucociliary transport is the lung's primary defense against noxious substances; however, the mucus cannot be too viscous or too thin for optimum transport. When the epithelial lining is damaged and inflammation occurs, both active ion transport and the mucociliary system are weakened. The bronchial goblet cells increase in size and number and cause more mucus to be formed. The mucus of asthmatic patients is thick, and mucus plugs are commonly found in the airways.

ASTHMA IS A COMPLEX DISEASE

Asthma is commonly seen in the feline and rarely seen in the canine patient. The cat with "feline asthma" may present as an acute emergency in severe respiratory distress or may have a more chronic history characterized by cough and wheezing. Acute feline asthma must be differentiated from symptoms associated with pleural effusion or pulmonary edema. Radiographs must be taken to assess treatment options and ascertain a diagnosis.

Asthma is a complex disease and is seen more often in pure-breds (Siamese, Persians) as opposed to mixed breed cats. Genetic variability contributes to a stronger immune system, and as with all diseases, the stronger the immune system, the healthier the pet.

I believe that atopy (inhalant allergy) is the strongest risk factor for the development of asthma. In pets with a genetic predisposition towards asthma, exposure to dust mites, mold, pollen, or other air particles may trigger symptoms. Both humans and pets benefit greatly from indoor air filters. Believe it nor not, indoor air pollution may exacerbate respiratory ailments. Tobacco smoke; dirty ventilation ducts or poor ventilation; oxides of nitrogen from gas appliances, heaters, or stoves; oil boilers; accumulation of pesticide residues; and other pollutants are all contributors. Exposure to formaldehyde vapors and other volatile compounds, aerosol mists, sulfites, peroxide dyes, artificial colors, detergents, sulfur compounds, and other chemicals commonly found around the house cause or worsen asthma.

For a long time, asthma was viewed primarily as a broncho-constrictive disorder. The airways narrow and contract too much, causing the wheezing and difficulty in breathing. This is called bronchial hyperresponsiveness (BHR). The constriction or spasms involve the smooth muscles lining the cartilage rings that help form the tracheobronchial tree. Medical treatments used are bronchodilators, which force open the airways.

Asthma is predominantly an inflammatory disorder in which airway constriction is just a symptom of underlying inflammation. Remember, in inflammatory disorders there is an imbalance between TH_1 lymphocytes and TH_2 lymphocytes, whereby the TH_1 cells are depressed while TH_2 cells are elevated. The TH_2 lymphocytes are involved in the stimulation of B-lymphocytes, which produce immunoglobulins. It has been shown that IL-5 secreted by TH_2 cells promotes the production of eosinophils, which are involved in allergic reactions.[2]

Inflammation is the response to tissue insult or injury. This is a natural biochemical process by which the body attempts to repair damaged tissue. Lymphocytes respond to the noxious substances by sending out various chemical signals (cytokines), which attract inflammatory cells to the areas affected. Phagocytes engulf and digest dead and damaged cells or foreign particles. White blood cells (eosinophils particularly) release their own "chemical weapons," a second wave of signals (histamine, leukotrienes) that cause congestion and swelling. Needed nutrients, cells, and other substances from blood vessels are released to perform waste disposal and lay a repair matrix. Excess mucus, a protective mechanism that is supposed to rid the area of debris and protect the tissues from further irritation, adds to the congestion.

Interference with the inflammatory process (cortisone, antihistamines) can result in incomplete repair and unresolved inflammation. Even large doses of ascorbic acid (synthetic vitamin C), which has some antihistaminic effects, can slow the healing process. Medications may control symptoms, but tissue repair may be impeded, leaving the tissues open to further repeated injury. A vicious cycle evolves with continuous inflammation, repeated injury, repeated interference, and nonresolution of tissue repair. Ultimately, this leads to deterioration of the mucous membrane and epithelial lining of the respiratory tract. This tenacious mucus is secreted, which plugs areas of the bronchi and bronchioles, so breathing during an asthmatic attack is like sucking mud through a straw. All of these consequences make breathing more difficult. The immune system mechanisms are increasingly stressed and may begin to fail. Prescribed drugs can be lifesaving and provide temporary relief of symptoms, but it appears they also accelerate the damage done to the airways.

Long-term use of anti-inflammatory drugs, primarily corticosteroids, interfere with the inflammatory process, which can cause elevated blood pressure, osteoporosis, diabetes, adrenal insufficiency, liver disease, kidney disease, infections, and even cancer.

The success of long-term treatment must include a natural raw food diet. Eliminating refined, altered, and processed foods brings benefits to any disease condition, since such items not only provide little if any nutritive value, but they also tend to deplete the body of nutrients and supply toxic by-products. Further, these "dead foods" may interfere with stages of inflammation and repair.

Bioflavonoids, a natural constituent of vitamin C complex, can benefit pets with allergies and asthma. Antispasmodic substances are found in fennel, red bell pepper, cabbage, carrot, currant, cranberry, eggplant, grapefruit, orange, tomato, and acerola berry, which are all high in vitamin C complex.

About 50 percent of human patients with acute asthma attacks have low serum magnesium. High dietary magnesium intake has been associated with better lung function in humans.[3] Magnesium relaxes the constricted muscles of the lung bronchioles, alleviating the wheezing and severity of asthma attacks. Foods rich in chlorophyll such as dark green leafy vegetables are excellent sources of magnesium as well as other important nutrients.

Dietary deficiency of selenium, which also lowers the selenium-dependent enzyme glutathione peroxidase, is associated with increased risk of asthma. Increasing serum selenium levels and platelet glutathione peroxidase activity improves symptoms.[4] Supplementation results in significant clinical improvement. Selenium is the trace mineral "activator" for the vitamin E complex, which protects the mucous membrane lining of the respiratory tract. Good sources are raw milk, raw eggs, whole grains, seeds, nuts, and green leafy vegetables.

There is an inverse association in humans between intake of vitamin A complex and the degree of lung airway obstruction. Low serum levels of retinol are related to low values of respiratory function. Vitamin A complex is important to inflammation and repair, and is known to play an essential role in the health and resilience of mucous membranes. It is obvious that vitamins A and E are needed for proper cellular differentiation. It is important to remember that cats must have preformed vitamin A, because they are unable to convert beta carotene to vitamin A.

Natural fatty acids, including the omega-3 group, also protect mucous membranes. Increased dietary ingestion of omega-3 fatty acids (flax seed, fish oil) reduces the risk of developing childhood asthma and reduces current asthmatic symptoms including airway hyperresponsiveness.[5]

On the other hand, ingesting high amounts of refined and altered vegetable oils (omega-6 group) can increase the severity of asthma. One consequence may be that these foods increase production of compounds that exacerbate mucous secretion and muscle contraction during asthma attack.

Vitamin C is especially important to the health of the lungs. It is the major antioxidant present in the lining of the airway surfaces.[6] High intake and high blood levels of vitamin C have been shown to protect against the development of chronic respiratory symptoms in humans. Remember, both dogs and cats are able to produce vitamin C—unlike man, primates, and guinea pigs. However, with disease and stress, it is helpful to give pets foods high in vitamin C complex. Lower intakes of vitamin C were significantly associated with lower values on pulmonary function and increased wheezing. Plasma, serum, and leukocyte (white blood cell) levels of vitamin C are often reduced in humans with bronchial asthma.[7] Administration of ascorbic acid (synthetic vitamin C fraction) sometimes brings pharmacological improvement, but often no changes are found. Taking large doses of ascorbic acid before exercising has helped some people prevent or postpone exercise-induced asthma (temporary drug response). Ascorbic acid acts as an antihistamine, thus exerting a mild antibronchospastic action, an inhibition of bronchial responsiveness. This also slows or inhibits the natural healing process. It is much more reasonable to ingest whole, complex, nutritional sources of vitamin C, which support inflammation, repair, and the general health and function of mucous membrane and smooth muscle. Healing is a slow relentless process, without a quick fix. Rather, food concentrates work slowly to get to the underlying cause and to balance biochemistry—not to stimulate or suppress an effect.

Typically, asthmatics show low levels of pyridoxine (vitamin B_6), which is needed to convert the amino acid tryptophan to niacinamide (vitamin B_3).[8] Theophylline, a bronchodilator used in respiratory diseases, has been shown to significantly depress the levels of the active form of B_6.[9] Other B-complex factors are also affected and needed for respiratory health. For example, the vitamin B-complex is involved in the production of nitric oxide, a needed vasodilator and inflammation mediator. All of the B vitamins and their coworkers are functionally inseparable, so this whole complex would assist in asthma, particularly in relation to the autonomic nervous system.

Supporting the health and repair (including inflammation) of the mucous membrane lining and other tissues of the respiratory tract as well as supporting the adrenal glands, thymus gland, lymphatic system, and other participating aspects of the immune response would only be prudent. Glandular supplements could be used, including lung, adrenal, and thymus substances. In short, all the vitamins, minerals, trace elements, amino acids, fatty acids, enzymes, and unknown nutrients in raw, live, unprocessed foods are needed for optimum health.

At Highlands Veterinary Hospital, a number of different modalities—acupuncture, nutrition, biological response modifiers, and herbs—are all used to cure asthmatic patients. I have found that the only way to affect a long-term cure is the use of a natural raw food diet and biological response modifiers (substances that rebalance the immune system).

HERBS USED IN ASTHMA

Coleus Forskohlii
Coleus, a member of the mint family, grows on dry hill slopes in India, Nepal, Sri Lanka, and Thailand.

Forskolin is believed to be the active compound; however, other components within the plant extract may enhance its absorption and activity. Forskolin has the unique ability to activate the enzyme adenylate cyclase, which increases levels of cyclic adenosine monophosphate (cAMP) in cells. Cyclic AMP is an important cell-regulating compound. This energy-rich compound activates numerous enzymes involved in various cellular functions.[10]

The physiological effects of a raised intracellular cAMP level include: inhibition of platelet activation and degranulation, inhibition of histamine release, increased force of contraction of heart muscle, relaxation of the arteries and other smooth muscles, increased insulin secretion, increased thyroid function, and increased breakdown of fat cells.

An important action of forskolin is the inhibition of platelet activating factor (PAF). It is well known that PAF plays an important role in many inflammatory and allergic processes.[11]

It is important to realize that allergic conditions such as asthma are characterized by a decrease in cAMP in the bronchial smooth muscle and skin respectively. As a result of this derangement, mast cells degranulate and smooth muscle cells contract. In addition, these allergic conditions are also characterized by excessive levels of PAF. Coleus may be particularly useful in asthma to increase cellular levels of cAMP, which relaxes bronchial muscles and relieves symptoms in asthma. Forskolin has been shown to have remarkable effects in relaxing constricted bronchial muscles in asthmatics.[12]

Cordyceps

In traditional Chinese medicine (TCM), it is said that cordyceps goes to the meridians of the kidneys and lungs. For centuries, cordyceps has been the medicine of choice in TCM for treating respiratory diseases. During modern times, doctors in China have prescribed cordyceps for chronic bronchitis, asthma, pulmonary and congestive heart disease, and tuberculosis. The use of cordyceps in the treatment of asthma may be due to its relaxant activity on the trachea. At the Meiji Institute of Health Science in

Japan in 1995, researchers found that an extract of cordyceps inhibited tracheal muscle contractions and relaxed the airways of rats. Interestingly, the cultured fungus (mycelial extract) was six times more potent than the wild fungus. They concluded that the extract of cordyceps seems to "facilitate the increase in the pulmonary ventilation during movement." Since the extract inhibited constriction of the trachea, it appears that the airways would have less resistance and more dilation from cordyceps.[13] I often use this herb in respiratory problems. Remember, it is also a potent biological response modifier as well.

Ephedra (Ma-huang)

Ephedrine is a chemical compound found in all species of ephedra, of which the Chinese varieties, known as ma-huang, are the most widely used in herbal medicine. Ephedrine's basic pharmacological action is similar to that of epinephrine (adrenaline), although ephedrine is much less active. Ephedrine stimulates both the alpha and beta receptors of the nervous system as well as induces release of norepinephrine, which further stimulates the nervous system. As a result, the central nervous system is activated, the metabolism is increased, and blood flow through the peripheral muscles is enhanced at the expense of kidney and intestinal blood flow.[14] Ephedrine relaxes the bronchial muscles, the muscles of the airways, and the muscles of the uterus.

I use ma-huang only in combination with other herbs. I have found that a little ma-huang goes a long way with synergistic effects when combined with appropriate herbs.

Ginkgo

Ginkgo contains several unique molecules known collectively as ginkgolides, which antagonize platelet activating factor (PAF), a key chemical mediator in asthma, inflammation, and allergies. Ginkgo is one of the more potent anti-asthmatic herbs I have used. In several double-blind studies, the anti-asthmatic effects of orally administered or inhaled ginkgolides have been shown to produce improvements in respiratory function and to reduce bronchial constriction.[15, 16]

Glutathione (Stabilized)

Humans with arthritis, diabetes, cardiovascular disease, lung disease, chronic renal failure, liver disease, neurologic disorders, and cancers have been found to have deficient levels of reduced glutathione.

Reduced glutathione is a tripeptide composed of the amino acids cysteine, glycine, and glutamic acid. Glutathione in the reduced form is made in every cell in the body. Being in the chemical form enables glutathione to donate electrons. The ability to donate electrons is what gives reduced glutathione its biological activity, as compared to oxidized glutathione, which has already donated electrons, and is no longer of any value.

Reduced glutathione neutralizes free radicals, which are highly reactive molecules that contribute to virtually every degenerative disease, including cancer and the aging process. Reduced glutathione is the most important antioxidant inside the cells and therefore plays a critical role in minimizing damage by free radicals.

I use a product called Recancostat, a stabilized reduced glutathione with anthocyanins, which are bioflavonoid plant pigments that vary in color from orange-red to blue-black. Remember, the best precursors to glutathione are raw milk and raw eggs.

Glycyrrhiza Glabra (Licorice)

Licorice root has a long history of use as an anti-inflammatory and anti-allergy agent. The primary active component of licorice root in this application is glycyrrhetinic acid, a component shown to have cortisol-like activity.[17] Licorice also has expectorant activity, which is useful in asthma. I use licorice on an as-needed basis for two to four weeks at a time to minimize water retention.

Lyprinol

Lyprinol is a natural extract of the New Zealand green-lipped mussel (perna canaliculus). This unique stabilized extract contains a rare form of fatty acids called tetraenoic acids. Fatty acids control the types and amounts of eicosanoids produced by the body. Eicosanoids such as leukotrienes and thromboxanes play a major part in inflammatory processes. The inflammatory process while normal and necessary can remain overactive due to excess levels of eicosanoid metabolites, leading to chronic inflammation. I have used lyprinol with success for a number of inflammatory processes in both dogs and cats. Lyprinol's stabilized lipid extract appears to down regulate proinflammatory eicosonoids such as leukotrienes.[18]

Magnolia Plus

This herbal formula consists of magnolia flower, angelica, ginkgo, ma-huang, tussilago, morus, perilla, scute, licorice, cimicifuga, silar, iridium, asarum, akebia, and pinellia. I formulated this herbal combination and have used it long term in both dogs and cats with remarkable success. Magnolia has been shown to have antibacterial, antifungal, and antiprotozoal effects. This herbal formula is versatile in most respiratory diseases and works quickly in alleviating mild to severe symptoms in asthma, bronchitis, or sinusitis.

Panax Ginseng

Chinese ginseng is quite versatile in its ability to normalize many body functions, including lung function. Ginseng is well known as an adaptagen. Studies on pulmonary function suggest that ginseng protects the lungs against free radical injury and may enhance vasodilatation of constricted lungs.[19] From personal experience, a hot ginseng tea with lemon and honey will quell a harsh cough within thirty minutes. Whenever I get a cold, I drink ginseng tea, which soothes my throat and lungs while enhancing my immune system.

Tylophora Asthmatica

Tylophora is used primarily in Ayurvedic (Indian) medicine for asthma and the treatment of respiratory tract disorders. It is believed that the alkaloids, especially tylophorine, inhibit the degranulation of mast cells, which prevents the release of many inflammatory mediators.[20]

CHRONIC CANINE BRONCHITIS

Bronchitis refers to an infection or inflammation of the bronchi (passageway from trachea to lungs), while pneumonia refers to infection of the lungs. Chronic bronchitis in dogs is poorly understood, and I suspect that there are several etiologies involved. All chronic respiratory diseases must have a thorough work-up to rule out potential bacterial, viral, or cardiac abnormalities. Chronic bronchitis and pulmonary fibrosis (scar tissues) are the most frequent causes of chronic coughing and shortness of breath in dogs.

In the acute and severe stage, the use of antibiotics and corticosteroid treatment reduces clinical signs markedly. Long-term treatments involve the use of biological response modifiers along with previously mentioned herbs in the asthma section of this book. Anecdotal reports relate the use of methyl-sulfonylmethane (MSM) to reduce scar tissue. Remember, a raw food diet, especially one including a natural source of vitamin A such as raw liver, cod liver oil, raw milk, butter, fish, and cheese, is important. Vitamin A is a potent biological response modifier and is essential for the health and integrity of mucous membranes.

SINUSITIS

Any factor that causes inflammation of the lining of the sinuses may result in partial obstruction and drainage with subsequent infection of the nasal passages. In puppies and kittens, viral, bacterial, and fungal infections must be ruled out, while in older animals, cancer also must be viewed as a possibility. Careful history may lead to a diagnosis.

Stray dogs with a thick greenish nasal discharge accompanied by a cough, elevated temperature, and hardened footpads should be viewed with a high suspicion of distemper. Many dogs that are rescued from animal shelters contract infectious tracheobronchitis or kennel cough, which is self-limiting and resolves in ten to fourteen days in most cases. Because of the self-limiting nature of this disease, treatment is indicated only in situations where the signs are severe and persistent. This disease is a combination of several viruses and bacteria. However, in young puppies with a fever and dry hacking cough, short-term antibiotics along with biological response modifiers shorten the course and prevent complications such as pneumonia.

Feline viral rhinotracheitis affects primarily the eyes and upper respiratory tract of cats. Symptoms may include sneezing, coughing, and nasal and ocular discharge with an accompanying fever. In most cases, particularly in older cats, the disease is self-limiting and no treatment is needed. However, in young kittens with a high fever, treatment with biological response modifiers and antibiotics is indicated. Antibiotics do not work on viruses; however, this disease lowers the immune system, which enables normal bacterial flora to overgrow and cause a secondary bacterial infection that has the potential to kill young kittens. Many kittens must be force-fed until their body temperature returns to normal. Nasal discharge may hinder their ability to smell food; so foods with stronger aromatic characteristics such as fish may entice cats to eat on their own.

Chronic sinusitis in dogs and cats has an underlying cause such as low immune function and pollen allergies. Many of these animals have secondary bacterial or fungal infections, which must be addressed with appropriate medicines. A combination of biological response modifiers, Magnolia Plus herbal combination, and acupuncture has cured many patients.

BACTERIAL PNEUMONIA

Bacterial pneumonia frequently occurs secondary to other disease. Predisposing diseases in the dog include megaesophagus, aspiration, airway foreign bodies, viral infections (canine distemper), and immune deficiency. Predisposing diseases in the cat include aspiration, airway foreign bodies, bite wounds, and viral infections such as feline leukemia virus (FELV), feline infectious peritonitis (FIP), and feline immunodeficiency virus (FIV). Thorough work-ups must be done and should include radiograph, blood work, and culture and sensitivity. Antibiotics must be instituted immediately and continued for ten to fourteen days past resolution of clinical and radiographic signs.

To expedite the healing process, I administer a raw food diet, biological response modifiers, and acupuncture. Many pet owners are taught coupage to help loosen secretions and encourage coughing. In this technique, the owner uses a cupped hand to gently tap the back and chest to loosen mucus from the lungs. This is a life-threatening situation and aggressive therapy must be instituted immediately to save the life of the patient. Frequent monitoring is important to assess response to treatment.

chapter 14

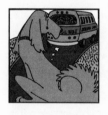

Herbal Help for Neurologic Disorders

NEUROLOGIC DISORDERS IN DOGS AND CATS ARE MANY AND HAVE VARIED CAUSES. We will briefly touch upon some of the more common problems seen in a small animal practice. Keep in mind that many disorders require a thorough history and laboratory work-up. Magnetic resonance imaging (MRI) is the most accurate tool for ruling out tumors of the central nervous system and is becoming more widely available. Lastly, when considering neurologic disorders, "behavioral problems" must be addressed and treated appropriately. Millions of animals are euthananized yearly due to "behavioral problems." Many pets can be saved with a little patience, some training, and medication. These pets are our family members and must be given our love and understanding.

CANINE SEPARATION ANXIETY

Canine separation anxiety is physiologically quite similar to anxiety in humans. Both humans and dogs are social animals. This perhaps is a key to their survival from ancient to modern times. The same physiological response to anxiety that can trouble modern humans and dogs saved their ancestors' lives. The anxiety that early humans felt while confronting the challenges of food on the hoof or avoiding being some other creature's dinner would trigger the release of hormones such as adrenaline. These hormones intensified focus and pumped up muscles, allowing early man to fight or flee when needed. Humans or dogs with built-up anxiety have built-up energy just ready to "explode" inappropriately.

Dogs with pathological anxiety (separation anxiety) are extremely stressed as they struggle to overcome their discomfort of being separated from their attachment figure (owner). Remember, dogs are descendants of wolves, which are highly social creatures. They greet us as a subordinate member of a pack. So, it is not surprising that dogs, being highly social creatures, form strong attachments to their owners, and that when their owner is absent, the dog experiences anxiety. Over time, the dog's anxiety level increases, triggering autonomic stimulation, which eventually results in outward expressions such as destructive behavior, urination, defecation, vocalization, or salivation when left alone.[1] Brain chemistry plays a significant role in the development and progression of separation anxiety.

It is easy for us to anthropomorphize, and say that the dog is "spiteful," "spoiled," or "angry" at us. However, it is more accurate to describe the dog's disruptive behavior as a distress response that occurs when the dog is left alone or separated from the person to whom it is attached. Canine separation anxiety is one of the most common behavioral disorders of dogs. It has been estimated that in the average veterinary practice in the U.S., up to 14 percent of canine patients exhibit one or more signs of separation anxiety.[2] Unfortunately, in the absence of successful training or treatment, the outcome for affected dogs usually involves relinquishment to a humane society or shelter, abandonment, or euthanasia.[3, 4]

How a dog responds to emotional situations depends on

neurotransmitters in the brain. Each neurotransmitter acts on a particular area in the brain and triggers specific responses. An increase or decrease in a certain neurotransmitter can affect mood, attitude, and/or activity. The five neurotransmitters that appear to be most affected by herbs or drugs are:

1. serotonin

2. norepinephrine

3. acetylcholine

4. dopamine

5. gamma-aminobutyric acid (GABA)

As two potent compounds responsible for emotions, serotonin and norepinephrine are considered to have a strong effect on how a dog reacts to certain emotional situations.

Serotonin is probably the most important neurotransmitter in the control of sleep, pain, aggression, sexual behavior, thermoregulation, and food intake. Serotonin also plays a significant role in fear and anxiety (low serotonin levels is the principle element in the fear mechanism), which is a key consideration in cases of canine separation anxiety. It has been shown that increased serotonin levels would reduce the distress and fear associated in dogs with separation anxiety.[5]

A safe Western drug approved for this disorder is clomicalm™ (clomipramine hydrochloride). I have used this drug successfully in a number of dogs with separation anxiety. I have also used clomipramine in other anxiety-related problems, such as relocating to a new house. Clomicalm is a triclyclic antidepressant. In general, tricyclic antidepressants appear to block the re-uptake of norepinephrine and serotonin from new synapses. Of all the tricyclic antidepressants on the market today, clomipramine is the most serotonin-selective, which results in an increase in the action of serotonin. Dogs receiving clomipramine have a decreased level of fear and anxiety and increased receptivity to behavioral modification or training. Clomipramine is safe and effective; an overdose may cause transient lethargy.

For other anxiety disorders such as traveling, I have used an herbal combination containing valarian, chamomile, kava kava, and St. John's wort. This herbal combination has been safe and effective in dogs and cats.

Chamomile

Chamomile is frequently used as a mild sedative to calm the nerves, reduce anxiety, and induce a state of relaxation without disruption of normal function or interfering with motor coordination. It has also been used to calm upset stomachs and ease digestion. Chamomile's effectiveness is also due to its anti-inflammatory properties, which help sooth ulcers and reduce gastritis and other mucous membrane inflammations.[6]

Kava Kava

Kava kava root has been used in the South Pacific for centuries as a relaxant herb. The active constituents consist of a group of lactones that are similar in structure to myristicin, which is found in nutmeg.[7]

Kava's exact mechanism of action on the central nervous system is still not fully understood. However, it is hypothesized that the kava lactones potentiate GABA receptors in the brain.[8] (GABA or gamma-amino butyric acid is a neurotransmitter.) Studies have shown that kava kava has both anticonvulsive and anxiolytic effects.[9, 10] I have also used this herbal combination to successfully reduce the dosage of phenobarbital in epileptic patients.

St. John's Wort (hypericum perforatum)

Farmers have long considered St. John's wort a nuisance plant because of its photosensitizing effect on cattle. Nevertheless, humans have used it for centuries for a wide variety of ailments, including nervous disorders, depression, neuralgia, wounds, burns, kidney problems, and for its antibacterial and anti-inflammatory actions.

Hypericum contains numerous biologically active constituents, including hypericin and its derivatives, hyperforin, flavonoids, catachin, and others. Since there are several compounds within St. John's wort extract, it has been difficult to study the precise way this herb works in relieving depression. Perhaps the combination of compounds has a synergistic therapeutic value, while individual ingredients would, on their own, have little effect. However, one can surmise that some of the ways this herb works is by influencing levels of chemicals within the brain, specifically dopamine, serotonin, and norepinephrine.

In a study done on rats, hypericum extract caused a 50 percent inhibition of serotonin uptake by rat brain cells.[11] Antidepressants such as Prozac and clomicalm work by inhibiting the re-uptake of serotonin. This is why they are called serotonin re-uptake inhibitors. As a beneficial consequence of these re-uptake inhibitors, more serotonin stays around to influence brain cells, and a happier mood is created.

Another way that hypericum and pharmaceutical antidepressants work is by inhibiting an enzyme called monoamine oxidase (MAO).[12] This enzyme degrades many brain chemicals, including serotonin, norepinephrine, epinephrine, and especially dopamine. By inhibiting this enzyme, more of these brain chemicals stay in the brain, leading to enhanced alertness and mood elevation. One well-known medicine, selegeline or deprenyl, works by inhibiting this enzyme. It is also known to elevate mood and cognitive ability of humans and animals.

Valerian (Valeriana Officinalis)

For many years, valerian has been used as an antispasmodic and sleep aid. Today, this herb is widely used throughout Europe as a mild sedative and sleep aid for insomnia.

The sedative effects of valerian root are attributed to the valepotriates, a group of unstable compounds whose degradation products also possess sedative activity.

Valerian works by enhancing the action of the neurotransmitter gamma-amino butyric acid (GABA), which in turn blocks the arousal of brain centers. Valium works in a similar way. In fact, valerian root exerts its action on the benzodiazepine (valium) receptor sites in the brain.[13] It is apparent that the complex mixture of chemicals have a synergistic effect to bring about the sedative action.

COGNITIVE DISORDERS

Canine cognitive dysfunction syndrome is similar to Alzheimer's disease in humans. As the brain ages, it goes through definite age-associated degenerative changes. It is generally believed, and research has shown, that cognitive ability in dogs tend to decline with age.[14] A common misunderstanding is that we are born with a fixed number of neurons, which then degenerate and become fewer with age; in essence, our brain function peaks in young adulthood, and it's all downhill from there and nothing can be done about it. This statement is not entirely correct.

While the number of neurons in the brain cannot be increased, we can increase the number of connections to the neurons, which makes the brain work better. Humans can certainly take up new hobbies and interests while increasing their physical activity. It is not so easy for our elderly canine companions. However, we can slowly increase their physical activity while at the same time increase mental stimulation by taking them out to new and different locations for walks or hikes. We can attempt to make their lives as enjoyable as possible, keeping in mind that many also have arthritic problems as well as visual and hearing impairments. Remember, stress, toxins, and dead devitalized food cause the brain to age quickly and to actually become smaller. Once cognitive dysfunction develops, it may not be reversible, but treatment can limit further degeneration. I have seen some dogs act like "puppies" according to their owners after a combination of treatments such as acupuncture, good nutrition, and neutraceuticals (discussed later). Just as in cancer, prevention is the best medicine. A considerable amount of research shows that degeneration of the brain is caused by three factors:

1. Poor nutrition (processed food).

2. Toxins (organic solvents, paint thinner, kerosene, petroleum).

3. Compromised blood supply to the brain.

This is a complex subject matter, and certainly more research is needed to delineate all of the ramifications involved. Certain pieces to the puzzle have been answered thus far. It has been shown that certain changes with neurotransmitters occur within the brain and are thought to play a role in cognitive dysfunction. These changes may include depletion or imbalance in levels of acetylcholine, serotonin, dopamine, and norepinephrine. Levels of monoamine oxidase B (MAO-B), an enzyme that catabolizes (breaks down) dopamine, have been found to increase in older animals and humans.[15] It is hypothesized that elevated MAO-B activity may result in decreased brain dopamine concentration and play a role in the development of canine cognitive dysfunction.

A neuro-toxin protein called beta amyloid accumulates in the cerebral cortex and hippocampus of the canine brain and forms plaques. Though no one knows why beta amyloid is deposited in the brains of older dogs, I suspect that it may be the overreactive activity of microglia cells in the brain. Microglia cells in the brain monitor the health of surrounding cells and become highly phagocytic if they detect injured cells. Older cells are more susceptible to free radical damage. Like the macrophages, they migrate to the site of injury and ingest pathogens, diseased cells, and other debris. Microglia cells, along with secreting growth factors, also secrete digestive enzymes that may damage brain cells. Microglia cells protect the brain from pathogens; however, as with other white blood cells, they tend to overreact to damage to ensure that all the pathogens are destroyed and cellular debris is removed. As can be imagined, uncontrolled or excessive activation of the microglia cells may result in degenerative brain disorders such as cognitive dysfunction or Alzheimer's disease in humans. This may be an autoimmune-like reaction to certain toxins, pathogens, and vaccines.

Because the brain is so metabolically active, it has tremendous need for a regular supply of micronutrients. It's not surprising that a deficiency of almost any nutrient can cause brain dysfunction. A raw natural diet during an entire lifetime not only slows degeneration of the brain, but will prevent 90 percent of all other diseases including cancer. Prevention is the best medicine and must always be our goal.

HELP FOR THE AGING BRAIN

CDP Choline (cytidine - 5' diphosphocholine)

It has become increasingly clear that phospholipids—the various fatty acid mineral molecules that comprise a significant portion of the membrane—play key roles in maintaining brain cell efficiency. Phospholipids can be likened to attendants at the entry gates of nerve cells (and all cells of the body); they help transport substances as fuel needed for healthy and efficient operation. Phospholipids maintain and regulate cell membrane integrity, strength, permeability, elasticity, and resistance to stress, among other functions. Without sufficient nutrients (Vitamin E complex) to properly maintain phospholipids, we would not be able to think very well.

More than thirty years of European brain research has resulted in knowledge of CDP choline, also known as citicoline, a naturally occurring precursor to one of the most important phospholipids, phosphatidylcholine. In addition to its role in neuron membrane structural function, phosphatidylcholine is thought to be valuable in lipid turnover and communication signaling among neurons. It also acts as a neuroprotector. CDP choline donates the components choline and cytidine (both needed for phosphatidylcholine synthesis) required to form, repair, and even restore function to nerve cell membranes. In addition, choline promotes the synthesis of acetylcholine, a neurotransmitter intimately associated with cognitive function. As an information-transmitting molecule, acetylcholine is necessary for proper memory function and is especially important for aging brains. Research has shown that in addition to promoting phospholipid synthesis, CDP choline also inhibits phospholipid degeneration.[16]

Researchers have isolated several interesting mechanisms by which CDP choline might work to improve cognitive function in human Alzheimer's patients. Alzheimer's disease (AD) patients were given 1,000 mg daily dose for a period of one month and were found to have slight improvements in mental performance.[17] Scientists noted reduced brain theta activity and increased alpha activity in specific regions of the brain. Theta activity is associated with mental lethargy, while alpha activity is connected to mental stimulation. There were also indications of CDP choline's favorable effects on the immune system.

Another interesting benefit of CDP choline is its apparent ability to help cognitive and motor deficits. When injected at a dose of 10 or 20 mg/kg/day for twenty days, twenty-four-month-old male rats showed enhanced learning memory capacity. Only one injection was needed to protect against behavioral alterations caused by amnesia-producing drugs. An improvement in motor performance and coordination were also observed in aged rats.[18] Other rat studies found no difference in the effects of CDP choline upon oral or intraperitoneal injections.[19] This demonstrates that it is well absorbed orally and not destroyed by gastrointestinal juices. A good natural source is raw egg yolk.

Deprenyl (Selegiline)

I have used deprenyl for canine cognitive dysfunction for ten years. My personal experience has been quite rewarding. Positive results are usually seen in less than a week, though some dogs take a month to benefit from deprenyl. It is safe, and I have not seen any side effects; however, an overdose can cause blood pressure elevation.

This drug was originally manufactured in a factory in Hungary where most of the research originated. I became aware of deprenyl after Joseph Knoll published a paper reporting that with deprenyl—known for its brain-protecting properties—he had more than doubled the remaining life expectancy of twenty-four-month-old rats.[20] A few years later, a Canadian group reported that the same dosage of deprenyl also had extended the remaining life expectancy of laboratory animals.[21] So, why would a substance that prevents dopamine breakdown and protect neurons result in extended youth or life span? A youthful brain may be the key to a youthful body. Always keep in mind that a natural raw food diet is important for health and longevity.

Currently, only the L-form of this drug is in widespread clinical use in humans and dogs. Deprenyl is used for its ability to inhibit the B form of monoamine oxidase (MAO), an enzyme that functions in the brain to break down neurotransmitters. The A form, MAO-A, is found in most neurons and is most effective for breaking down the neurotransmitters serotonin, adrenaline, and noradrenaline. MAO-B, by contrast, is found in non-neuron brain cells and is more effective in breaking down the neurotransmitter dopamine. Drugs that inhibit MAO-A are used as antidepressants, whereas drugs that inhibit MAO-B are more effective as treatments for cognitive dysfunction.

Deprenyl can protect brain cells in many ways. The first and most obvious is through the inhibition of MAO-B. More than 80 percent of the dopamine in the brain is in the basal ganglia. MAO-B in the basal ganglia is almost completely inhibited by deprenyl. MAO-B inhibition reduces degradation of phenylethylamine even more effectively than it inhibits dopamine degradation. Phenylethylamine stimulates release of dopamine and serotonin, in addition to acting as a direct stimulant on dopamine receptors.

It's important to realize that the breakdown products of dopamine resulting from MAO-B degradation are hydrogen peroxide, ammonia, and an aldehyde. These are highly toxic and reactive compounds that contribute to brain degeneration and free radical reactions.

Besides causing MAO-B inhibition, deprenyl can increase the formation of the natural antioxidant enzymes super oxide dismutase (SOD) and catalase in the substantia nigra, striatum, and cerebral cortex regions of the brain. Knoll believes that it is this effect of deprenyl, rather than MAO-B inhibition, that results in life span extension.[22] It's important to note that rat brains metabolize dopamine differently than either humans or dogs. Most deprenyl life span studies have been conducted on rats whose brains use MAO-A, rather than MAO-B, to metabolize dopamine. Thus, inhibition of MAO-B metabolism of dopamine seems unlikely to be the mechanism of extended rat's life span. It appears that the potent antioxidant activity of dopamine is responsible for life extension in rats.

One intriguing piece of research shows deprenyl increases cell levels of the natural antioxidant enzyme superoxide dismutase by direct alteration of gene/protein transcription/synthesis. By acting directly on DNA, deprenyl also increases nerve growth factors and halts the death of cells and other proteins involved in protecting brain cells.[23]

Ginkgo

Ginkgo has become one of the most popular dietary supplements in the world. There are now more than 1,000 published studies about ginkgo, some that indicate that this potent flavonoid may have antiaging effects throughout the body. It has powerful therapeutic properties for the treatment of a number of serious medical conditions, including cognitive dysfunction, asthma, allergies, canine vestibular syndrome, cerebrovascular insufficiency, and circulatory disorders. Ginkgo has been used in traditional Chinese medicine for thousands of years.

The main reason why ginkgo biloba has such a broad variety of effects on the body is that it makes the whole circulatory system more efficient. By improving both the elasticity and tone of the blood vessels, it enhances blood flow. Ginkgo is unique because it affects all parts of the circulatory system, arteries, veins, and capillaries, and is therefore called a trivasoregulator (able to harmonize the total function of the circulation). A healthy circulatory system will provide nutrients including oxygen to all parts of the body and thus improve its function. This is particularly critical in the brain, where the cells are extremely susceptible to a lack of oxygen (hypoxia). It extends the ability of brain cells to withstand periods of oxygen deprivation, thus making it useful in treating strokes. Ginkgo protects small blood vessels against spasm and loss of tone, has a relaxing effect on the vessel wall, and protects capillaries from becoming fragile or leaking blood into tissues. It also acts to prevent the abnormal development of blood clots inside arteries and veins. I have seen dogs with conditions such as cerebrovascular accidents or mini strokes respond rapidly to ginkgo's effects.

In humans, clinical uses of ginkgo have included the treatment of early stroke, senility, and radiation-induced brain edema. Other disorders that have benefited from ginkgo include vertigo, deafness, embolism, and some eye disorders, including macular degeneration and diabetic vascular disease. Ginkgo has brought about strategically significant increases in alertness and mental responsiveness in healthy people, especially at higher doses. For example, in a study of 216 patients who were treated for twenty-four weeks with 240 mg a day of ginkgo extract or placebo, the patients receiving ginkgo improved on tests assessing attention, memory, behavior, and activities of daily life.[24]

Standardized ginkgo extract is a highly refined compound produced from the leaves, nuts, and branches of the ginkgo tree. Pharmaceutical-grade ginkgo consists of 24 percent flavonoid glycosides (supposedly for optimum therapeutic effects) and at least 6 percent of the terpenes ginkgolides A, B, and C and bilobalides. The flavonglycosides, which are part of the bioflavonoid family, are flavonoid molecules that are unique to ginkgo. Recently the Japanese have developed a new extraction process whereby they have been able to assay ginkgo extract at 28 percent glycosides and 7 percent terpenes. This new extract may have more beneficial effects than the old standard 24 percent extract. A comparison study of the two extracts would be important for both human and veterinary patients.

It is interesting that the mixture of biologically active natural products gives the entire extract a complex range of activity. For example, the flavonoids act as a free radical scavenger, while the terpenes, particularly ginkgolide B, interfere with or block the action of platelet activating factor. (PAF has been implicated in asthma, allergies, immune disorders, etc.) Both free radical formation and PAF can disrupt vascular membranes, resulting in increased vascular permeability, which in turn is associated with the impairment of cerebral blood flow seen particularly in elderly humans and dogs.

Ginkgo biloba extract appears to delay mental deterioration during the early states of Alzheimer's disease. In fact, ginkgo biloba extract may help reverse some of the disabilities associated with Alzheimer's and help the human patient maintain a normal life without having to be hospitalized. Geriatric dogs can benefit from ginkgo's ability to delay mental deterioration as well as increase circulation to other parts of the body (heart, kidney, legs).

Ginkgo biloba is unique in its capacity to simultaneously reduce vascular spasm in one area and restore tone in another area when needed. This is an extremely beneficial feature that vasodilating drugs lack.

Huperzine A

Huperzine A is a natural compound isolated from the club moss, huperzia serrata. It has been used in China for centuries to improve memory, focus, and concentration, especially among the elderly. It is well known that memory loss or impairments and cognitive dysfunctions are accompanied by a reduction in acetylcholine synthesis and/or release in the nerve cells.[25] This has led to research into the usage of synthetic and natural compounds for Alzheimer's disease in humans. Unfortunately, many drugs have a narrow safety range and must be used with caution.

Huperzine A is a potent anticholinesterase inhibitor. Acetylcholine is a neurotransmitter in the brain that is responsible for carrying electrical impulses from one nerve to another. It is made in the end section of nerve fibers and packaged into small vessels where it is stored until released. Once acetylcholine has been secreted by the nerve ending, it persists for a few seconds. In a normal brain, the enzyme acetycholinesterase serves a "clean-up" function by breaking down the acetylcholine, splitting it into an acetate molecule and choline. The choline is then transmitted back into the nerve ending to be used again to make acetylcholine. The brains of humans and presumably dogs with cognitive dysfunction demonstrate a deficiency of acetylcholine because of damage to the nerve cells that secrete it. Even with this deficiency, the acetycholinesterase enzyme keeps working to get rid of whatever acetylcholine is released from the damaged nerve cell. This creates a deficiency. Huperzine A stops this enzyme from breaking down acetylcholine, thus preventing deficiency and improving mental function. This herb is safe and, when used along with other natural cognitive enhancing modalities, offers a brighter future for humans and animals.

Phosphatidylserine (PS)

Phosphatidylserine plays a major role in determining the integrity and fluidity of brain cell membranes. Membranes are the cells' major work surfaces, and nerve cells especially depend on membranes to carry out their specialized functions. As part of the membrane, PS helps eliminate wastes and improve intercellular communications, cellular movement, and ion transport.

Normally, the brain can manufacture sufficient levels of PS, but if there is a deficiency of B-complex vitamins (folic acid and B_{12}) or of essential fatty acids, the brain may not be able to make sufficient PS. It has been shown that low levels of phosphatidylserine in the brains of elderly humans impairs mental function, while supplementation enhances brain function.[26]

Vinpocetine

Vinpocetine, a pharmaceutical extract from the periwinkle plant, has been used in Europe as a "smart drug" since the 1970s. It has been used for the treatment of cerebrovascular disorders and symptoms related to senility in humans.

Vinpocetine functions via several important mechanisms to correct multiple known causes of aging. It is well established that normal aging results in a reduction of blood flow to the brain and a decrease in the metabolic activity of brain cells. The biological actions of vinpocetine initially showed that it enhances circulation and oxygen utilization in the brain, increases tolerance of the brain toward diminished blood flow, and inhibits abnormal platelet aggregation that can interfere with circulation or cause a stroke.[27, 28] In addition to more efficient cerebral microcirculation, vinpocetine has been found to increase brain cell energy through its effect on ATP (cellular energy molecule) production. Vinpocetine also increases the brain's ability to function through more efficient utilization of glucose and oxygen while at the same time providing increased protection against ischemia (diminished blood flow). Since many brain disorders have been found to be caused by poor circulation, neuronal damage due to lack of oxygen, and insufficient amounts of energy, it makes sense that anything that helps brain function in these ways would also help memory and cognitive function. This is a safe herbal extract that I have used in both dogs and cats with encouraging results.

Interestingly, the molecular evidence indicates that the neuroprotective action of vinpocetine is related to its ability to maintain brain cell electrical conductivity and to protect against damage caused by excessive intracellular release of calcium. Vinpocetine apparently enhances cyclic GMP levels in the vascular smooth muscle, leading to reduced resistance of cerebral vessels and increased cerebral blood flow.[29] Vinpocetine possesses a mechanism that improves blood flow by inhibiting phosphodiesterase enzyme that degrades cyclic GMP. The degradation of cyclic GMP causes arterial constriction and reduced blood flow.

EPILEPSY

The terms epilepsy and seizures are used interchangeably by many specialists. However, I prefer to define epilepsy as a disorder of recurrent seizures with no underlying process, while seizures have a known underlying cause (such as brain tumor). The precise electrophysiologic and molecular mechanisms that underlie seizures are poorly understood. What we do know is that seizures are linked to membrane potentials, ionic fluxes, and generation of action potentials. In the brain, the neurons' action potentials result from changes in the membrane permeability to sodium, chloride, calcium, and potassium. As the action potential reaches the axon terminal, calcium channels allow entry of calcium ion into the terminal, causing the release of a neurotransmitter. These are normal populations of cells firing at a rhythmic and repetitive manner. Seizures occur when there is an imbalance between the excitation and inhibition of these cells.[30] This is certainly a simplistic rendition of a seizure but an important one.

When a pet exhibits seizures, it is important to take a complete history. For example, many puppies of the miniature breed types have seizures due to hypoglycemia. They must have access to a high protein diet at all times. If they go into seizure, they must be given karo syrup immediately. However, other pets may need to have complete blood work-up, urinalysis, cerebral spine fluid analysis, radiographs, and even MRIs to diagnose brain lesions.

Figure 14.1

Causes of Seizures

- Hypothyroidism (↓ thyroid)
- Hypoglycemia (↓ glucose)
- Hypoxia (↓ oxygen)
- Hepatoencephalopathy (liver disorder)
- Hypocalcemia (↓ calcium)
- Electrolyte Imbalance
- Brain Tumors
- Meningitis/Encephalitis
  - Distemper, FIP, FELV
  - Bacteria
  - Fungi (Cryptococcis)
  - Protozoa (Toxoplasmosis, Neospora Caninum)
- Hydrocephalus
- Toxins
  - Permethrins in Cats
  - Organophosphates
  - Heavy Metals
  - Herbicides and Pesticides
  - Plants (amanita mushroom)
- Vaccine Reactions

This is only the tip of the iceberg as to the causes of seizures. One must be a detective when dealing with seizures to confer appropriate treatments.

Standard Western therapy for epilepsy is the use of drugs such as potassium bromide, phenobarbital, and various valium-type drugs.

In treating seizures, I have had tremendous success with the use of acupuncture and a Chinese herbal combination known as Gastrodia and Uncaria, which is composed of gastrodia, gambir, holiotis, scute achyranthes, eucommia, loranthus, motherwort, Fu-Shen, gardenia, and polygonum. How exactly this herbal formula works is not totally understood; however, the main active ingredient, gastrodia, is composed of various chemicals including vanillin, which has been shown to have anticonvulsive effects.[31]

Pets with neurologic diseases, in particular, need foods that are high in B-complex vitamins. For example, thiamine (B_1) is required for normal functioning of all body cells, especially nerves. A deficiency can prone a patient to neuritis, muscular weakness, dizziness, and mental confusion. Good sources of thiamin include raw organ meats, wheat germ, pork, whole grains, fish, nutritional yeast, raw milk, nuts, and oysters. Thiamin plays an important role in nerve conduction or transmission by potentiating the effects of acetylcholine, a compound formed from choline, which has many functions including conductor of the nerve impulse. Thiamin is concentrated in the protective myelin sheaths of nerve fibers; this is one area where acetylcholine is made. Synthetic thiamin is potentially dangerous, and an overdose can result in convulsions, weakness, neuromuscular paralysis, and anaphylactic shock. Veterinarians must not inject synthetic B-complex vitamins into the intravenous fluid bags of critically ill patients. This will further put a strain on the detoxification mechanism of the already compromised patient. Remember, a natural raw food diet—and not processed foods that come in a bag or can—is where to get all the known (and unknown) B-complex vitamins. Remember, vitamin B_4, also known as the antiparalytic factor, is required for the normal development and function of human and animal brains.[32, 33]

SPINAL DISORDERS

All spinal cord diseases are dangerous and potentially lethal. A complete neurologic exam, radiographs, and even magnetic resonance imaging (MRI) are employed to differentiate various problems. Weakness in the hind limbs may indicate arthritis of the spine and hips, disc herniation, neoplasms, spinal embolism, metabolic or endocrine abnormalities, and degenerative myelopathy.

Intervertebral Disc Disease

Intervertebral disc disease is a common disease encountered in dogs and is often associated with severe pain and/or neurologic dysfunction. Clinical signs may include pain, ataxia paresis, and paralysis. In severe cases, deep pain perception to the hind limb may be lost on palpation. The most common area of spinal dysfunction is where the thoracic and lumbar vertebral canals meet.

Certain breeds are at high risk for this disease. It is quite obvious and unfortunate that short-legged and long-backed breeds known as chondrodystrophoid breeds (dachshund, Lhasa apso, beagle) are genetically predisposed to this disorder. In these breeds, the disc undergoes degeneration at a much earlier age than in other breeds. In degeneration, the softer spongy part of the disc calcifies. These degenerative changes develop when the animal is young (only several months in age), but clinical signs of the disease may not appear until three to seven years of age.

Treatment and management of these patients in veterinary medicine is controversial. Western medicine will usually institute corticosteroids and surgery at the first sign of intervertebral disc disease. I believe that 90 percent of these patients do not need and should never undergo surgery. I have had excellent results with the use of acupuncture and herbs. In an acute situation, I will inject DMSO intravenously, instead of corticosteroids. DMSO is safe with no known side effects. It has potent antioxidant effects as well as some analgesic activity. Helpful neutraceuticals include arthred, New Zealand green-lipped mussel, methylsulfonylmethane (MSM), glucosamine sulfate, ginkgo, and stabilized glutathione. Physical therapy treatment, in which the pet is allowed to swim in a pool or a bathtub along with massage, is helpful.

Degenerative Myelopathy

Degenerative myelopathy is a degeneration of the spinal cord that occurs predominantly in German shepherds or German shepherd cross-breeds.[34] The age range of affected dogs that I have seen runs from five to fourteen years. There certainly appears to be a genetic predisposition, as it is rarely seen in other breeds.

Keep in mind that many of these dogs may be concurrently afflicted with arthritic hips, which will further exacerbate the problem. Initially, the patient may show signs of hind limb ataxia, knuckling of the toes, wearing of the nails of the digits of the rear paws, and stumbling, as if in a drunken state. With time, signs worsen and progress to paralysis and eventual death. At times, afflicted dogs will develop urinary and fecal incontinence. Fortunately, pain is not an issue with this disease.

The diagnosis of degenerative myelopathy is based on exclusion of other diseases. It is suspected in any German shepherd or cross with progressive spinal ataxia and weakness. It is important to rule out other diseases such as spinal neoplasia, disc disease, lumbosacral stenosis, spinal embolism, and peripheral neuropathy. At times magnetic resonance imaging (MRI) must be employed to rule out other diseases.

It is unfortunate, but no definitive cause or cure has been found for this disease. A variety of different treatment modalities have been tried with little or no success. Some of the treatments range from acupuncture, DMSO, steroids, immunomodulators, myelin, various herbs, and aminocaproic acid. Some researchers believe that aminocaproic acid stabilizes or slows the progression of the disease. I have found it to be of some benefit in a few patients. I believe that this is an autoimmune disease. Interestingly, a number of my patients were afflicted with parvovirus as puppies. Perhaps the virus or subsequent vaccinations triggered an immune response. Certainly, more basic research is needed as to the cause, so that prevention can be instituted in this breed of dog.

Knowledge in the treatment of this disease may come from an unlikely source. Research in the treatment of humans with Alzheimer's disease may benefit dogs with spinal cord diseases as well as degenerative myelopathy. For the past forty years, Dr. Harry S. Goldsmith has been conducting research into Alzheimer's disease. The treatment involves placing a part of the body known as the "omentum" directly onto the brain or spinal cord with its attached blood supply. The omentum is a packet of fat and blood vessels lying over the intestines like a blanket. Goldsmith found that he could use the omentum to provoke new blood vessels to grow in areas of the body lacking blood flow.[35-38] In 1999, Goldsmith reported on a patient who was transposed with the omentum thirteen years after a stroke. The patient's neurologic function improved and was maintained.[39] In 1986, Goldsmith reported that he had isolated an angiogenic (blood vessel promoting) factor from the omentum. One injection causes new blood vessels to sprout.[40] The omentum is a fatty hunk of tissue that not only provokes angiogenesis, but also increases choline acetyltransferase, the enzyme that catalyzes the reaction that creates acetylcholine in the brain. This can certainly benefit humans and animals with brain damage as well.

Perhaps the most important aspect of the omentum is the fact that it has an abundance of nerves. Those nerves, just like the ones in the brain, need nourishment and support. The omentum has an ability to generate neurochemicals that nourish nerves and help them grow. One of them, fibroblast growth factor (FGF),[41] has been shown to provoke the growth of new brain cells in areas of the brain affected by Alzheimer's diseases and potentially areas of degenerated spinal cord. In short, when omental tissue is transposed to the brain or spinal cord, the brain or spinal cord may benefit from a new influx of growth factors. It is time that this form of basic research is done in the veterinary community, at the university level, so that more help and hope can be given to these dogs that are part of our families. Perhaps the best medicine lies within ourselves and not with the drug companies.

chapter 15

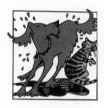

Good Nutrition Prevents Cancer

No OTHER MEDICAL DIAGNOSIS STRIKES AS MUCH FEAR IN THE HEARTS OF PEOPLE AS THE DIAGNOSIS OF CANCER. It is a disease that has affected most of us, either directly or indirectly through relatives or friends. It is also a major killer in our pet population. Statistics are unreliable; however, in one study 45 percent of dogs that lived to ten years or older died of cancer.[1] Statistics in humans indicate that one in four will contract cancer.

Cancer is a disease process in which healthy cells stop functioning and maturing properly. A mishap occurs inside malignant cells. It is important to note that no one insult will cause cancer; rather, it is the result of a number of insults over time. Usually a number of years are required to develop cancer. Perhaps it begins with a change (mutation) on the genetic blueprint (DNA). The altered DNA makes copies of itself and passes its information and gene sequences on to other cells, which then become cancer-prone. As the normal cycle of cell creation and death is interrupted, the newly mutated cancer cells begin multiplying uncontrollably, no longer operating as an integrated and harmonious part of the body. Cancer represents an accelerated process of inappropriate, uncontrolled cell growth. Cancer, despite its horror for the individual, is a natural phenomenon, and it represents the body's response to a continuous attack on its balancing regulatory mechanisms over time. I emphasize this, because a carcinogen ingested once will never cause cancer. The majority of cancers seen in animals are in animals over ten years of age.

Cancers are divided into five major groups for both humans and animals.

1. **Carcinomas** form in the epithelial cells that cover the surface of skin, mouth, nose, throat, lung airways, genitourinary, and gastrointestinal tracts, or that line glands such as the breast or thyroid. Lung, breast, prostate, skin, stomach, and colon cancers are called carcinomas and are solid tumors.

2. **Sarcomas** are those that form in the bones and soft connective and supportive tissues surrounding organs and tissues, such as cartilage, muscles, tendons, fat, and the outer linings of the lungs, abdomen, heart, central nervous system, and blood vessels. Sarcomas are solid tumors, but are highly malignant and the most deadly.

3. **Leukemias** form in the blood and bone marrow; these abnormal white blood cells then travel through the bloodstream creating problems in the spleen and other tissues. These are not solid tumors.

4. **Lymphomas** are cancers of the lymph glands. Lymph glands act as a filter for the body's impurities and are concentrated in the neck, groin, armpits, spleen, center of the chest, back of knees, pre-scapula, and around the intestines. Lymphomas are usually made up of abnormal lymphocytes (white blood cells) that congregate in the lymph glands to produce solid masses.

5. **Myelomas** are rare tumors that arise in the antibody-pro-
ducing plasma cells or hemopoietic (blood cell producing) cells in various tissues in the bone marrow.

Compared to normal cells, cancer cells have prolonged life
spans. It is ironic, given that cancer can potentially prove fatal to
its host and thus to itself as an unwelcome parasite. They are essentially immortal, but on a suicide mission. Not only do cancer
cells not die when they are supposed to, they also fail to develop
the specialized functions of their normal counterparts. A tumor
may become like a parasite and develop its own network of blood
vessels to siphon nourishment away from the body's main blood
supply. It may also secrete toxins, which further weaken the host.
I have noticed that surgical excision of benign tumors improved
the pet's well-being and quality of life. If the tumor invades adja-
cent normal tissue or spreads through lymph vessels or the blood
vessels to other normal tissues, the tumor is considered malignant. Most cancer victims do not die from the initial multiplica-
tion of these abnormal cells, but as a result of this secondary
process called metastasis.

A common term used in oncology is differentiation. Differentiation is a process by which unspecialized cells mature and become specialized to carry out specific tasks. Differentiated cells,
red blood cells for example, have a preset life expectancy and are
programmed to live, die, and be replaced on a precise schedule.
In cancer, there is an abnormal control over the way in which a
cell becomes specialized. Generally, a poorly differentiated cancer, in which the tumor cells bear almost no resemblance to normal cells of that particular tissue, is the most virulent and
dangerous. Tumors that are moderately differentiated generally
pose a more favorable outcome, with survival likely. A well-dif-
ferentiated cancer, though less common than a moderately differentiated one, can be nonmalignant. Remember, a cancer cell is
a once normal cell that cannot stop growing and multiplying. Most
cancer researchers believe that the cause of this behavior lies in

the genes of the cells.[2] This may or may not be entirely true. We must look at the whole being: cancer can only develop in an already diseased animal. Healthy humans or animals will *not* get cancer. In fact, it has been shown that a disturbance of the regulatory mechanisms and functions, as well as metabolism are demonstrable before the tumor itself appears.[3] Conditions have to be conducive for cancer to develop. Many checks and balances must fail over time for cancer to develop.

It seems that dysfunctions in the developmental processes of cells are at the heart of the cancer dilemma. Cells are apparently the most sensitive to the effects of carcinogens during the developmental period. On the other hand, cells are less susceptible to cancer as they age and become more differentiated, probably because they are no longer capable of dividing. Every body, whether human or animal, is constantly sloughing off old, used-up cells (catabolism), and producing new, mature cells (anabolism). Cellular replacement takes place at various rates, depending on the tissue or organ. Tissues that live in the gastrointestinal (GI) tract and skin cells, for example, experience a rapid cell turnover, while tissues such as the heart muscle and neurons of the central nervous system do not undergo significant or quick cell replacement. Cancers are more common in areas of faster cell turnover such as the skin and GI tract; they are more rare in the heart and central nervous system, where there is slow cell replacement.

FREE RADICALS: A CHAIN REACTION OF DESTRUCTION

Little was known about free radicals until about forty years ago. Today they are considered a major component in aging, disease progression, and, of course, cancer. Free radicals can be produced by external factors, such as radiation and toxins, as well as internal factors such as products of aerobic cellular respiration, immune cell activity, inflammation, and other processes. In humans, up to 5 percent of the oxygen taken in is converted to free radicals.[4]

Free radicals are molecules that contain an odd number of electrons. As such, they have a strong tendency to react with the electrons of other molecules. When a free radical contacts electrons of a stable molecule, the radical gains or loses electrons to achieve stability. However, this process disturbs the electron balance of the stable molecule, thereby creating a new free radical. In this way, free radicals initiate a chain reaction of destruction. It is a vicious cycle.

Free radicals are a natural by-product of everyday reactions that produce energy for the body. The energy is produced by reactions between many substances and oxygen. Without energy production, the body cannot survive. Think of the serious impairment to life that chronic fatigue syndrome causes with its malfunctioning energy production.

To counteract free radical damage, the body maintains a variety of antioxidants as a multilevel defense system. These include super oxide desmutase (SOD), catalase, and glutathione peroxidase. Other important nutrients are vitamins A, C, and E; selenium; zinc; and carotenoids. For example, macrophages and neutrophils destroy foreign microbes by producing what is known as a "respiratory burst" of hydrogen peroxide and free radicals. To prevent self-inflicted damage, macrophages contain high amounts of vitamin C.

Antioxidant defenses are not perfect, and DNA is damaged regularly. It has been estimated that there are 10,000 oxidative hits to DNA per cell per day in humans.[5]

The vast majority of these lesions are repaired by cellular enzymes. Those that are not repaired may progress toward neoplasia. Due to continual bombardment of DNA and other tissues by free radicals, the body must obtain ample antioxidant supplies through the diet. These include vitamins, flavonoids, and other compounds found in fresh fruits and vegetables.

Many pet foods are laced with various cancer-causing chemicals such as preservatives, pesticides, hormones, and herbicides. Couple this with contaminated water and our pets are constantly being assaulted by chemicals that the body must detoxify. (For information on detoxification, see chapter 10.)

THE TERRAIN IS EVERYTHING

Before Louis Pasteur died, he pronounced, "I have been wrong. The germ is nothing. The terrain is everything." What this means is that a healthy body cannot get cancer or succumb to infections. For example, a smoker, after years of tobacco use, may develop bronchitis; the linings of the respiratory tract have become unhealthy, irritated, and diseased. Eventually coughing, expectoration, and deterioration give way to decaying tissue and cancer. The decaying tissue can no longer reproduce normal cells, and the cellular environment can no longer cope with the chemical onslaught. The terrain is diseased. In humans, it has been estimated that the average cancer is present thirty-nine months before the patient or doctor discovers it.[6]

In the 1930s, Royal Rife proved that by altering the environment a harmless bacteria, virus, or fungus will revert to a virulent one.[7] In Rife's studies, the microbes were able to adapt to the environment and change as needed, depending on the media used. Pleomorphism, as this is called, is controversial and is not widely accepted by Western scientists. Research has since demonstrated in the laboratory that bacillus can change in size and take on the characteristics of a virus. The environment in which the microbes live provides the waste material, which they feed on or metabolize. The characteristics of the microbes are determined by what they ingest (deteriorating cells or toxins), and these in turn determine their virulence. Scientists have concluded that it is the toxic degenerative condition of the environment that causes cancer—not the microbe. However, viruses have been implicated in cancer.

There are some 70,000 chemicals in the environment, of which some 20,000 are known carcinogens.[8] Each year billions of pounds of pesticides are sprayed on crops for food, 90 billion pounds of toxic waste are dumped in thousands of toxic waste sites, and 9 million pounds of antibiotics are given to our farm animals to help them gain weight faster. Plus, there is an unknown amount of electromagnetic radiation. It is not surprising that one in three or four Americans will get cancer. There is evidence that dogs that live in a household in which the owners applied 2,4-D herbicides to their lawns have a higher incidence of lymphoma.[9]

Unfortunately, many fruits and vegetables that are essential to good health are contaminated with toxic chemicals including pesticides and industrial waste. These substances are often neurotoxic and carcinogenic. Even low doses over a prolonged period of time will cause cancer. The twelve fruits and vegetables that were found to contain the most toxic pesticides are: strawberries, green and red bell peppers, spinach, cherries, peaches, cantaloupe (Mexican), celery, apples, apricots, green beans, grapes, and cucumbers. Quite alarmingly, even previously banned pesticides were detected at high levels. The answer is to buy only organically grown fruits and vegetables and to wash them thoroughly.

THE ONCOGENE THEORY

Is there a gene, called an "oncogene," that causes cancer? It is thought that normal cells contain genes that are considered to cause cancer when they malfunction. Unfortunately, research using normal cells in vitro are not always reliable. As is true of all cell clones, these cells have an abnormal number of chromosomes, and chromosomal defects or mutations are seen in malignant cells. So inserting "oncogenes" into normal cell lines and observing the outcome may lead to a dubious conclusion. Cell line research is not always reliable because these cells, whether normal or cancerous, are easily disturbed.

Sometimes science is stranger than fiction; however, in the case of the oncogene theory, I believe it is all fiction. The oncogene theory presumes that cancer is caused by about twenty specific genes called "proto-oncogenes." It is theorized that hundreds of millions of years ago, some unique genes were incorporated into several types of viruses when the viruses infected cells. Supposedly, each of these genes gradually evolved into a "viral oncogene," which can initiate cancer when certain animals are infected by the virus. These same genes, staying behind in the cells of our early ancestors, evolved in a different way. Now they have normal functions in our cells and are referred to as proto-oncogenes. These proto-oncogenes are presumed to be normal parent forms of oncogenes. Theoretically—and this is not proven—if they are altered or mutated, they are transformed into oncogenes.

Cultured cell lines are fragile and mutate easily, and even altering the nutrients in the culture can cause alterations in the cells and cancer-like transformations. In fact, an article in the prestigious journal *Science* states that the chromosomes are riddled with weak points, known as fragile sites, that break or appear to form gaps easily, at least in cell lab culture.[10] I believe mutations are not the cause of cancer, but they are more likely the result of cancer. Cancer causes mutations. If cancer was caused by mutated genes, then the germ cells (sperm and ova) should also contain these altered genes. Every sperm and ova must contain these inherited genes. In humans with breast and ovarian cancers, it was shown that the relationship to most cancers by genetic transfer is unlikely and indirect at best.[11]

A WEAKENED IMMUNE SYSTEM IS RIPE FOR CANCER

Dr. Josef Issels echoes my thoughts when he says, "The development and dissemination of cancer becomes possible by the weakening or loss of the body's natural resistance." When the immune response, the body's defense system, is weakened, it cannot engulf and destroy abnormal or cancer cells or prevent them from multiplying. Such natural resistance is incapacitated as a consequence of the complex summation of noxious substances and damage, which has occurred some time before any sign or symptom of cancer appears. These noxious substances lead to a complex chronic metabolic disturbance and prepare the soil for what I have described as a "tumor milieu."[12]

Once again, the compromised biological terrain allows cancer to take hold and flourish. The toxic overload and the constant unrelenting assault on Mother Earth must stop for the cancer epidemic to reverse. Toxins not only cause DNA breakage, which can trigger cancer, but they also subdue the immune system, which then allows cancer to become the fox in the chicken coop, with no controlling force. To prevent cancer, we first must start with detoxifying Mother Earth. We must stop pollution at all levels and preserve our oceans, lakes, rivers, mountains, forests, and deserts; we must find biological control of pests while enforcing more humane farming practices. The dairy industry must be allowed to bring back certified raw milk. At present, only California and Georgia are legally allowed to produce certified raw milk. I drink nourishing and wholesome raw milk daily and have not gotten ill; on the contrary, raw certified milk is practically a perfect food. It has more than thirty enzymes, is palatable and a complete protein, and is high in omega-3 fatty acids; vitamins A, B-complex, C, D, and E; and many trace elements and minerals. Pets with serious illness respond quickly to the nutrients from certified raw milk. It is a myth that people will become ill from raw milk; on the contrary, more people have become ill from pasteurized milk.

NUTRITION AND CANCER

All cancer treatments must start with good nutrition. A raw natural food diet is imperative to good health. All processed foods must be eliminated. If a food will not rot or sprout, then do not buy it. The cells of the body have similar biochemical needs to a bacteria or yeast cell. Foods that have a shelf life of a millennia are not going to nourish a body. If bacteria or fungi are not interested in a food, then what makes you think that your pet's body is interested? If it comes in a paper bag or can, then it is "dead." "Live" foods deteriorate and rot over time. Life begets life.

Do not be fooled by synthetic vitamins in pill form. These are drugs, and the body recognizes them as such. In fact, I believe that synthetic vitamins put more of a strain on the body. Synthetic vitamins are foreign to the body and not natural (as nutrients from food are) and must be detoxified out of the body. Remember how bright your urine appears when ingesting ascorbic acid. This will not occur when ingesting real vitamin C from fruits and vegetables. Vitamins from natural foods have a synergistic effect, and only they can heal, prevent, and conquer cancer.

There are many anticancer agents in plant foods, including more than five hundred mixed carotenoids, more than six hundred various bioflavonoids, lutein, lycopenes, and canthoxanthin. The important point is that there are many unknown nutrients in foods that are yet to be discovered. Raw meats with all of their inherent live enzymes and nutrients are essential to combat cancer. A study in Holland of colon cancer and meats found no link whatsoever between the condition and the consumption of red meats, animal fat, or animal protein.[13] Perhaps the meat in Holland has less poison residue. Red meat is a healthy food for your dog and cat. If possible, purchase free-range chickens and eggs and meat from pasture-fed cattle. Lamb and turkey also contain important nutrients, as do whole grains and nutritional yeast. See chapter 5 for more details on natural foods.

This is but the tip of the iceberg on biological response modifiers, and it is also important to review adjunctive cancer treatment. Herbs with anti-inflammatory effects such as curcumin, flax, licorice, and quercetin have also been shown to have antineoplastic effects.

COMMON CANCERS IN DOGS AND CATS

There are more than a hundred cancers recognized in dogs and cats. We will discuss a few of the most common. It is important to realize that cancer cells produce noxious substances (prostaglandins) that suppress the immune system.

Tumors

Tumors of the skin and subcutaneous tissue are commonly seen in dogs. One tumor I see quite often is mast cell tumors. These are aggressive tumors with the potential for recurrence and metastasis. I have treated them successfully with surgery, nutrition, and a variety of biological response modifiers (substances that balance the immune system). Chemotherapy is ineffective, though frequently used in veterinary medicine. Radiation therapy may be employed depending on the location (proximity to vital organs). The pets I have treated have done well, without the side effects of chemotherapy.

Osteosarcomas

Osteosarcomas are the most common primary bone tumors seen in dogs. Bone cancer in cats is extremely rare. These tumors must be differentiated from osteomyelitis (infection) and fungal infections. Frequently biopsies must be performed to ascertain a diagnosis. Osteosarcomas are often seen in large breed dogs in the long bones. Amputation is frequently used; however, Colorado State University is experimenting with limb-sparing surgical techniques. Here again I have used various biological response modifiers in conjunction with amputation. Dogs can function well with three limbs and even live happy, content lives. Once again, chemotherapy is not recommended, though it is frequently employed in veterinary medicine. The agents used to treat bone cancer are extremely toxic and frequently will lead to the demise of the pet much sooner than from the cancer itself. Cisplatin or carboplatin are two agents frequently used to treat bone cancer; I believe both will destroy the pet due to kidney failure much sooner than osteosarcoma. Interestingly, in a survey of seventy-nine Canadian oncologists, all of them would encourage patients with nonsmall cell lung cancer to participate in a chemotherapy protocol, yet 58 percent said that they themselves would not participate in such a therapy and 81 percent said that they would not take cisplatin under any circumstances.[14]

Lymphomas and Leukemias

Canine lymphomas and leukemias are treated well with chemotherapy. This is the only cancer that I treat with chemotherapy, along with herbs and nutrition. Though side effects do occur, most dogs tolerate chemotherapy much better than humans. I have seen various survival statistics that range from two months to two years, though some pets actually become cured. Pets must be monitored closely while on chemotherapy, because bone marrow suppression may occur. The herbs complement chemotherapy quite well and give the pet a better chance for long-term survival while minimizing side effects. Gleevec, a new human cancer drug, may be helpful to pets in the future. Unfortunately, it is extremely expensive at this time (about $18.00 a capsule).

Mammary Cancers

To prevent mammary cancers, female dogs must be spayed before the first heat period. Neutering male dogs will prevent testicular tumors, perianal adenomas, as well as prostate disease. It is much better to prevent cancer than to treat it.

Tumors of the Intestinal Tract

Tumors of the intestinal tract are seen with increasing frequency in veterinary medicine. This is probably due to various toxins in processed food. The most common treatment is surgical resection. I also use a healthy diet and biological response modifiers.

Bladder Cancer

In recent years, I have seen an increase in bladder cancers in the canine patient. These tumors are transitional cell carcinomas with the potential to recur and metastasize. Surgery is the treatment of choice when possible. I use herbs, nutrition, and have included cyclooxygenase-2 (COX-2) inhibitor (Etodolac) as adjunctive therapy. Many types of cancer cells produce excess amounts of COX-2 and use this as a biological fuel to stimulate their rapid division. The theory for cancer patients using COX-2-inhibitors is to deny the COX-2 enzyme to cancer cells.[15] Interestingly, curcumin, an Indian herb, has been shown to have anti-inflammatory, antioxidant, and COX-2 inhibiting effects. This may explain why it has been successfully used in cancer patients.

Etodolac, also known as Etogesic, is widely used for canine arthritic patients. It is a safe drug, and many dogs get relief for their arthritis as well as inhibition of cancer growth. Etodolac has the potential to be used in a number of deadly cancers such as colon, pancreas, breast, lung, bladder, head, neck, and others. I would like to see research in this area. Many other herbs, such as boswellia, ginger, feverfew, and Chinese skull cap, have shown COX-2 inhibition.

Spleenic Hemangiosarcomas

Spleenic hemangiosarcomas are perhaps the most lethal of the canine cancers. Some of the signs may include acute anemia, listlessness, enlarged abdomen, and sudden collapse. Hemangiosarcomas of the spleen are quite friable and bleed readily. The patient is at risk of death from an acute hemorrhagic crisis. As soon as the patient is stabilized, spleenectomy must be performed. Most patients will survive the surgical procedure but are at an increased risk for metastasis within a few months. I have successfully added biological response modifiers, herbs, and raw food diets, and have seen cures with this dreaded disease. Although chemotherapy is routinely administered in veterinary medicine, I do not believe chemotherapy is rewarding for this cancer. Again, review the list under the biological response modifiers and allergic and immune-mediated diseases in chapter 6.

With cancer treatments, there are no magic bullets. We use multiple treatments and substances working together synergisticly to affect major changes in the cancer process, from containment, to remission, to a happy and health life that is cancer-free. Synergy in alternative medicine treatments means many substances working cooperatively in such a way as to enhance the overall effect, creating a stronger defense than single substances could ever produce alone.

ADJUNCTIVE TREATMENTS USED IN CANCER PATIENTS

Carnivora®
Carnivora® is a phytonutrient supplement made from the pressed juices of the entire dionaea muscipula (Venus flytrap) developed by German physician Dr. Helmut Keller. It is widely used in cancer treatments in Germany and is the subject of considerable research. The main immunomodulating phytochemical is plumbagin and its analog.[16]

Together plumbagin and its analog (hydroplumbagin) provide a variety of pharmacological properties, including antitumor, antibacterial, antiviral, and antiprotozoal activities.

A primary mechanism of action of the digestive juices produced by the Venus flytrap is the inhibition of protein-kinases. Tumor cells require protein-kinases (enzymes) to synthesize proteins. By blocking protein-kinases, the cancer cells are inhibited and die.[17]

Immune stimulating and modulating effects are shown in the rebalancing of CD4/CD8 ratio (helper T cells to suppressor T cells) with the ingestion of Carnivora.® Other documented effects are increased debris clearance as well as increased activity and proliferation of macrophages, granulocytes, total T-lymphocytes, and natural killer cells.[18] I use Carnivora® in solid tumors but not in lymphomas or leukemias.

Enzyme Therapy
The body's immune system does not normally react to its own cells. However, when a cell becomes cancerous, antigens form on the cell's surface. The immune system may then identify these cells as foreign and destroy them. However, even a healthy immune

system cannot always destroy all cancer cells. It is believed that tumors are covered by a fibrin coating on the surface, making it difficult for the body to identify them.[19]

In a healthy body, certain proteolytic enzymes strip away the fibrin that protects cancer cells from detection. This paves the way for cancer cell destruction by the immune system. The more cancer cells the body produces, the more enzymes the body needs. It is believed that the depletion of endogenous enzymes may allow cancer cells to flourish.

As mentioned earlier, with healthy pets there is a balance between cancer cell production and cancer cell destruction. As pets age, injuries and illness place added stress and strain, and the body cannot produce sufficient proteolytic enzymes to help break down and eliminate cancer cells. Therefore, enzyme supplementation is essential. Enzymes also enhance the immune system.

I prefer to use Wobenzyme imported from Germany. It is composed of pancreatin, trypsin, chymotrypsin, bromelain, papain, and rutin (bioflavonoid) and is entericly coated to be absorbed in the small intestines and, therefore, absorbed in the blood.

Essiac

For a period of almost sixty years, Rene Caisse, a nurse living in Canada, treated hundreds of people with an herbal remedy she called Essiac (Caisse spelled backwards). She discovered this remedy through a patient in the hospital where she worked. The patient claimed an herbal remedy given to her by an Ajibwa Indian herbalist cured her cancer.

The Essiac formula consists of Indian rhubarb, sheephead sorrel, slippery elm, and burdock root. Many companies have since modified it and added cat's claw, kelp, blessed thistle, red clover, and watercress.

According to a report issued in 1993, Essiac strengthens the immune system, reduces toxic side effects of many drugs, increases energy level, and has anti-inflammatory effects.[20] Studies of some of Essiac's components (burdock, Indian rhubarb, shepherd sorrel, slippery elm) have demonstrated a significant amount of anticancer activity.[21] For example emodin, one of the main constituents in rhubarb, has been shown to inhibit various cancer cell lines and to reduce tumor cell numbers and increase survival time in leukemic mice.[22, 23] Japanese researchers have identified a potent factor in burdock that can block cell mutation.[24]

No hard scientific evidence exists that Essiac is effective; however, hundreds of anecdotal reports do. I have been using Essiac as an adjunct, along with many other herbs and biological response modifiers, with success. I found Essiac to also be an effective liver detoxifying remedy. It is safe in both dogs and cats and comes in tea and capsule forms. Buyers must be wary, as there are many inferior forms of this tea.

Lapacho (Pau D'rco)

Lapacho has been used for at least a thousand years by Brazilian Indians. Its use has spread from Brazil to other parts of South America. The bark has been used as a poultice for treating skin diseases such as eczema, psoriasis, fungal infections, and skin cancer. Many people have used the tea from the bark as a blood purifier, while the inner bark has been favored in treatments for diarrhea, fever, sore throat, wounds, snakebites, and carcinomas.[25]

The main active constituent is lapachol, a substance that has been studied by the U.S. National Cancer Institute. Unfortunately, most lapacho products in the marketplace are devoid of lapachol or are of inferior quality. I use a lapacho product from Paraguay, which appears to be more efficacious than the products I have used from Brazil.

Nine human patients with various cancers (liver, kidney, breast, and prostate adenocarcinomas and squamous cell carcinoma of the palate and uterine cervix) were given pure lapachol with meals. All nine patients showed a shrinkage of tumors and reduction in tumor-related pain, three patients experienced complete remissions, and there were no adverse side effects.[26]

Lapacho products need standardization and certainly more

scientific research. I have used lapacho in many immune-compromised pets with great success. I have also been impressed by its antifungal effects.

Pacific Yew

Research with the Pacific yew tree started in the 1960s. By 1966, researchers were able to isolate a particular compound from the bark of the tree, which appeared to have anticancer properties. The Pacific yew cancer-killing compound was named "taxol" (taken from the tree's Latin name taxus brevifolia).

Historically, various Native Americans used the Pacific yew tree to cure skin diseases, stomach and lung problems, wounds, kidney problems, colds, fever, and arthritis, and to alleviate pain in childbirth.[27]

Unlike other species of yew around the world, the Pacific yew does not contain levels of compounds called taxines that make other species of yew toxic. This is why Native Americans and wildlife in the Pacific Northwest have been able to ingest Pacific yew for centuries without harm. Research has also shown that the Pacific yew is a rich source of beneficial phytochemicals (taxanes) that are unique to the North American variety.

The Pacific yew taxanes have unique anticancer mechanisms of action. Cancer cells replicate by sending out what are referred to as spindle fibers. At the end of these fibers, a new cancer cell forms. When the new cancer cell matures, the spindle fiber, which connects it to its parent cell, disintegrates. The new cell becomes separate and able to create more cancer cells. The process creates uncontrolled cell growth, which forms tumors and radically interferes with normal body function.

Most chemotherapeutic agents work by destroying the cancer cell's ability to form the spindle fibers (microtubules), which allow for cancer cell reproduction. However, the microtubules may grow back when the drug is stopped. The Pacific yew taxanes destroy cancer cells by a completely different mechanism. The taxanes allow the cancer cell to grow its microtubules, but then prevent the microtubules from disintegrating, which stops cell division and permanently stops the growth of cancer cells.[28]

Some herbs are beneficial when standardized; however, in the case of Pacific yew, the sum of the whole is better than the individual parts. When we use whole plants rather than isolated plant compounds, we get small amounts of many beneficial substances that do not overwhelm the body. We also get a full range of plant compounds such as lignins and flavonoids, which possess anti-inflammatory, antiviral, and antioxidant effects.

I have found the Pacific yew to be a promising adjunct to cancer therapy. Remember, synergism between many therapeutic modalities is the answer in cancer treatments.

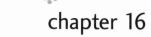

chapter 16

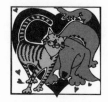

Putting It All Together

MODERN VETERINARY MEDICINE AS WELL AS HUMAN MEDICINE IS GROWING DAILY BY LEAPS AND BOUNDS with new diagnostic and therapeutic techniques. We should all be thankful that modern medicine is available for acute life-threatening situations. However, it is even more imperative to understand that at least 90 percent of all diseases seen in both humans and their pets are avoidable. It is immensely more preferable to avoid disease than to have to treat it after the fact.

We must all strive to ingest and feed our pets organically grown raw natural foods. Minimize processed foods as much as possible. Various herbs and biological response modifiers are gifts from nature, and we should learn to respect and use them.

In the last two to three hundred years with the advent of the modern Industrial Revolution, we have been poisoning mother earth along with the plants and animals that share her. Mankind's health as well as the health of all who inhabit this planet is dependent upon man's wise or foolish decisions. We should all strive to cleanse, detoxify, and allow mother earth to heal. And in return, we and our pets will heal as well.

In recent times, much research has involved the mind-body relationship of healing. In 1996, I went to China to study an ancient form of energetic healing called QiGong (pronounced chee-gong). In this form of healing, a QiGong master or healer emits energy with the intent to heal a patient. Like most Western-trained doctors, I was skeptical of this healing technique. However, since my initial exposure to QiGong, I have witnessed and experienced interesting energetic healings. We all possess energy and have the potential to cultivate and harness this energy within us. With practice, we all have the ability to cultivate this energy (Qi) with the intent to heal our pets and family members.

With life-threatening diseases, it is important to be optimistic and visualize the cancer destroyed, kidneys healed, or any other disease normalized. For example, with a cat in renal failure, place your hands on the back just above where the kidneys lie. Next, visualize a beam of light energy being emitted from the palms of your hands to your cat's kidneys. Visualize the light energy increasing circulation and blood supply, thus allowing the kidneys to regenerate and heal.

I have studied QiGong with many powerful Chinese masters in the United States, and I can tell you that it has literally changed my life and my outlook on the body's ability to heal. No matter how devastating the disease, this is always helpful adjunctive therapy. Remember, our pets heal us daily just by their presence, the least we can do is the same for them in time of need. Perhaps the greatest medicine lies within us.

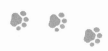

endnotes

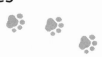

CHAPTER 1

1. J. Bland, *Functional Medicine: Understanding the Basics* (Gig Harbor, USA: Health Comm, 1995).

CHAPTER 2

1. Animal Protection Institute of America, *Investigative Report: Pet Food* (1996).

2. James G. Morris and Quinton R. Rogers, "Assessment of the Nutritional Adequacy of Pet Foods Through the Life Cycle," *Journal of Nutrition* (1994): 124.

3. Richard H. Pitcairn, D.V.M., Ph.D., and Susan Hubble Pitcairn, *Dr. Pitcairn's Complete Guide to Natural Health for Dogs and Cats* (1995).

4. M. Murray, *Encyclopedia of Nutritional Supplements* (1996).

5. Phillips Raudebush, D.V.M, "Pet Food Additives," *JAVMA* 203 (1993): 1667-70.

6. Ruth Winters, M.S., *A Consumer's Dictionary of Food Additives* (New York: Crown, 1994).

7. James Cargill, M.A., M.B.A., M.S., and Susan Thorpe-Vargas, M.S., "Feed That Dog! Part VI," *Dog World* (December 1993).

8. Ibid.

9. Animal Protection Institute of America, *Investigative Report: Pet Food* (1996).

10. Lisa Newman, "What's in Your Pet's Food?" *Tucson and Phoenix: Holistic Animal Care* (1994).

CHAPTER 3

1. J. De Cava, *The Real Truth About Vitamins and Antioxidants* (1997).

2. Elizabeth Somer, M.A., *The Essential Guide to Vitamins and Minerals* (New York: Harper-Collins Publishers, 1992).

3. R.L. Gross and P.M. Newbeme, *Physiological Review* 60 (1980): 188-302.

4. R.L. Wysong, *Rationale for Animal Nutrition* (1993).

5. Royal Lee, "What Is a Vitamin?" *Applied Trophology* (1956).

6. R.P. Murray, "What Is a Vitamin?" Manual, Biomedical Healer Foundation, Inc. (1993).

7. A. Grollman, "Anti-hypertension Factor in Vitamin A Complex," *Journal of Pharmacological and Experimental Therapy* 84 (1945).

8. T. Frieden, A. Sowell, and et al., "Vitamin A levels and severity of measles," *American Journal of Diseases in Children* 146 (1992): 182-86.

9. Krause and Mahan, *Food, Nutrition and Diet Therapy* (Nutrition Almanac, 1989).

10. M.D. Richards, "Imbalance of Vitamin B Factors," *British Medical Journal* (March 31, 1945): 4394-98.

11. *Scandinavian Veterinary* 30 (1940): 1121-43, cited in *Prevention Method for Better Health*, ed. J.I. Rodale (Rodale Books, 1968).

12. R.P. Murray, "Natural versus Synthetic," *Biomedical Nitty-Gritty* 3, no. 1 (1982).

13. G.B. Forbes, "Potatoes: A Reliable Source of Vitamin C," *Nutrition Today* 28, no. 1 (1993).

14. D. Schardt, "Grading Vitamin C," *Nutrition Action Health Letter* 21, no. 9 (1994).

15. P. Long, "The Power of Vitamin C," *Health* (October 1992): 67-72.

16. T. Brody, *Nutritional Biochemistry* (Academic Press, 1994).

17. D. Williams, *Alternatives* 3, no. 21 (1991).

18. Bicknell & Prescott, *Vitamins in Medicine* (1939).

19. Lester Packer, "Protective Role in Vitamin E in Biological Systems," *Am. J. of Clinical Nutrition* 53, no. 4 (1991).

20. Gullickson and Calverley, "Vitamin E. vs. Wheat Germ Oil," *Am. J. of Digest Disease* 12 (1945): 20-21.

21. *The American Journal of Clinical Nutrition* 53, no. 7 (January 1991), cited in *Alternatives* 3, no. 21 (1991): 2.

22. W.E. Shute, et al., *Alpha Tocopherol in Cardiovascular Disease* (Shute Foundation for Medical Research, 1952).

23. S. Azers and R. Mihan, "Vitamin E," *Southern Medical Journal* 67 (1974): 1308-12.

24. B. Liebman, "The Heart Health—E Vitamin?" *Nutrition Action Health Letter* 21, no. 1 (January–February 1994): 8.

25. C.E. Cross, "Oxygen Radicals and Human Diseases," *Ann. Intern. Med.* 107 (1987): 526-45.

26. R.R. Watson and T.K. Leonard, "Selenium and Vitamin A, E and C: Nutrients with Cancer Prevention Properties," *J. Am. Diet Assoc.* 86 (1986): 505-10.

27. K.N. Prasad and J. Edwards-Prasad, "Effects of Tocopherol (Vitamin E) Acid Succinate on Morphological Alterations and Growth Inhibition in Melanoma Cells in Culture," *Cancer Res.* 42 (1982): 550-55.

28. B.N. Ames, M.K. Shigenaga, and T.M. Hagen, "Oxidants, Antioxidants, and the Degenerative Diseases of Aging," *Proc. Nat. Acad. Sci.* 90 (1993): 7915-22.

29. D. Harman, "Free Radical Theory of Aging: The Free Radical Disease," *Age* 7 (1984): 111-13.

30. Meydani Metal. "Effects of Vitamin E Supplementation on Immune Responsiveness of the Aged" *Ann. NY Acad. Sci.* 570 (1989): 283-90.

31. A. Bjorneboe, et al., "Absorption, Transport and Distribution of Vitamin E," *J. Nutr.* 120 (1990): 233-42.

32. Lee. *Journal of Nutrition* 34 (1947): 571-79.

33. J.W. Simpson, et al., *Clinical Nutrition of the Dog and Cat* (1993).

34. R. Suskind, "Immunologic Mechanisms and the Role of Nutrition," in *Principals and Practices of Environmental Medicine* (1992).

35. R. Semba, et al., "Depressed immune response to tetanus in children with vitamin deficiency," *J. Nuts* 122 (1992): 101-7.

36. J.A. Levy, "Nutrition and the Immune System," in *Basic and Clinical Immunology*, 4th ed. (1982).

37. E. Seifter, et al., "Thymotropic action of vitamin A," *Fed Prac* 32 (1972): 947.

38. D.R. Campbell, M.D. Gross, M.C. Martini, G.A. Granditis, J.L. Slavin, and J.D. Potter, "Plasma Carotenoids as Biomarkers of Vegetable and Fruit Intake," *Cancer Epidemiol., Biomarkers and Prev.* 3 (1994): 394-500.

39. D.I. Thurmham, "Carotenoids: Functions and Fallacies," *Proc. Nutr. Soc.* 53 (1994): 77-87.

40. R.A. Jacob and B.J. Burri, "Oxidative Damage and Defense," *Am. J. Clin. Nutr.* 63 (1996): 9855-9905.

41. C.E. Cross, "Oxygen Radicals and Human Disease," *Am. Intern. Med.* 107 (1987): 526-45.

42. C.L. Rock, R.A. Jacob, and P.E. Bowen, update on "Biological Characteristics of the Antioxidant," *J. Am. Diet Assoc.* 96 (1996): 693-702.

43. A. Bendich, "Beta-carotine and the immune response," *Proc. Nutr. Soc.* 50 (1991): 263-74.

44. M. Alexander, H. Newmark, and R.G. Miller, "Oral beta-carotene can increase the number of OKT4+ cells in human blood," *Immunal. Letters* 9 (1985): 221-24.

45. P.R. Polan, M.S. Mikhail, J. Basin, and S.L. Romney, "Plasma Levels of Antioxidant Beta-carotene and Alpha-Topopheral in Literine Cervical Dysplasia and Cancer," *Nut. Cancer* 15 (1991): 13-20.

46. E. Negri, C. La Vecchia, S. Granceschi, F. Levi, and F. Parazzini, "Intake of Selected Micronutrients and the Risk of Endometrial Carcinoma," *Cancer* 77 (1996): 917-23.

47. S.T. Mayne, D.T. Janerich, and Greenwald. "Dietary Beta-carotene and Lung Cancer Risk in U.S. Nonsmokers," *J. Nat. Cancer Inst.* 86 (1994): 33-38.

48. Connett, et al., "Relationship Between Carotenoids and Cancer, The Multiple Risk Factor Intervention Trial Study," *Cancer* 64 (1989): 126-34.

49. D.A. Hughes, "Anti-Cancer Mechanism of Beta-carotene," *Journal of Lab. and Clin. Med.* (1997).

50. A.R. Mangles, et al., "Carotenoids Content of Fruits and Vegetables: An Evaluation of Analytic Data," *JADA* 93 (1993): 284-256.

51. S.T. Jung, Y.Y. Lee, S. Pakkala, and S. Devas, "1,25 (OH) (2)-16 ene-vitamin, D-3 in a potent antileukemic agent with low potential to cause hypercalcemia," *Leukemia Research* 18, no. 6 (June 1994): 453-63.

52. S. Nayeri, C. Danielsson, L. Binderup, and C. Carberg, "The anti-proliferative effect of vitamin D-3, analogues is not medicated by inhibition of the AP-1 pathway, but may be related to promoter selectivity," *ancogene* 11, no. 9 (November 2, 1995): 1853-58.

53. M.F. Holich, "Noncalcemic actions of 1,25-dihydroxyi vitamin D-3 and clinical application," *Bone* 17, no. 2 Suppl (August 1995): 107-111.

54. M. Murray, *Encyclopedia of Nutritional Supplements* (1996).

55. Animal Protection Institute of America, *Investigative Report: Pet Food* (1996).

56. H. Skalka and J. Prachal, "Cataracts and riboflavin deficiency," *Am. J. Clin. Nutr.* 34 (1981): 861- 63.

57. L.P. Case, D.P. Carey, and D.A. Hirakawa, *Canine and Feline Nutrition: A Sourcebook for Companion Animal Professionals* (St. Louis: Mosby, 1995).

58. M. Murray, *Encyclopedia of Nutritional Supplements* (1996).

59. J.R. DiPalma and W.S. Thayer, "Use of niacin as a drug," *Annual Review Nutrition* 11 (1991): 169-87.

60. E. Prien and S. Gershoff, "Magnesium oxide-pyridoxine therapy for recurrent calcium oxalate calculi," *J. Aral.* 112 (1974): 509-12.

61. S. Sarig, R. Azoury, and N. Garti, "Biological control to diminish dangers of urolithiosis," *Clin. Int.* 40 (1985): 274-76.

62. M. Murray, *Encyclopedia of Nutritional Supplements* (1996).

63. L.G. Hochmen, et al., "Brittle nails: Response to daily biotin supplementation," *Cutis* 51 (1993): 303-307.

64. L.B. Bailey, *Folate in Health and Disease* (New York: Marcel Dekker, 1995).

65. M.M. Werler, S. Shapiro, and A.A. Mitchell, "Periconceptional fabric acid exposure and risk of occurrent neural tube defects," *JAMA* 269 (1993): 1257-61.

66. D.J. Canty and S.H. Zeisel, "Lecithin and choline in human health and disease," *Nutri. Reviews* 52 (1994): 327-39.

67. R. Wurtman, A. Barbeau, and J. Growdon, "Choline and lecithium in brain disorders," *Nutrition and the Brain* Vol. 5 (New York: Raven Press, 1979).

68. G. Rosenberg and K.L. David, "The use of cholinergic precursors in neuropsychiatric diseases," *Am. J. Clin. Nutr.* 36 (1982): 708-20.

69. K. Okuda, K. Yashima, and T. Kitaazak, "Intestinal absorption and concurrent chemical changes of methylcobanin," *J. Lab. Clin. Med.* 81 (1973): 557-67.

70. M.I. Shevell and D. Rosenblatt, "The neurology of Cobalamin," *Can. J. Neurology Sci.* 19 (1992): 472-86.

71. M.A. Jolaludin, "Methylcobalamin treatment of Bell's palsy," *Methods Find Exp. Clin. Pharmacal.* 17 (1995): 539-44.

72. B.A. Yoqub and Siddigua, "Effects of methylcobalamin on diabetic neuropathy," *Clin. Neural. Neuropsy.* 94 (1992): 105-111.

73. K. Nelsson, et al., "Plasma homocysteine in relationship to serum cobalamin and blood folate in a psycho geriatric population," *Eur. J. Clin. Invest.* 24 (1994): 600-606.

74. Van Goor, et al., "Cobalamin deficiency and mental impairment in elderly people," *Age Review* 24 (1995): 536-42.

75. Y. Yao, et al., "Decline of sense cobalamin levels with increasing age among geriatric outpatients," *Arc. Fam. Med.* 3 (1994): 918-22.

76. E. Reynolds, "Multiple sclerosis and vitamin B12 metabolism," *J. Neuro-immuno.* 40 (1992): 225-30.

CHAPTER 4

1. Stewart, R.E., "Technology of Agriculture," *Encyclopedia Britannica* 15th ed. (1977).

2. Bergner, P., *The Healing Power of Minerals, Special Nutrients and Trace Elements* (Prima, 1997).

3. Harris, R.S., "Affects of agricultural practices on the composition of foods," in R.S. Harris and E. Karmos, ed., *Nutritional Evaluation of Food Processing* 2nd ed. (Westport, CT: 1975).

4. Ensminger, A. H., et al., *Food and Nutrition Encyclopedia* (Clovis, CA: Pegus Press, 1983).

5. Hall, R.H., *Food for Thought: The Decline in Nutrition* (New York: Harper and Row, 1976).

6. Ingham, E.R., "Interactions between invertebrates and fungi: Effects on nutrient availability," in G.C. Carrol and D.T. Wicklaw, ed., *The Fungal Community: Its Organization and Role in the Ecosystem* 2nd ed. (New York: Marcel Dekker, 1992): 669-90.

7. Coleman, D.C.; Odum, E.P.; and Crossby, D.A., "Soil biology, soil ecology and global change," *Biol. Fert. Soils.* (1992).

8. U.S. Department of Agriculture, Agricultural Research Service, "Composition of Foods: Raw, Processed, Prepared," *Agriculture Handbook No. 8* (1963).

9. U.S. Department of Agriculture, Agriculture Research Service, *Nutrient Database, SR11* (1997).

10. U.S. Department of Agriculture, Agricultural Research Service, "Composition of Foods: Raw, Processed, Prepared," *Agriculture Handbook No. 8* (1963).

11. U.S. Department of Agriculture, Agriculture Research Service, *Nutrient Database, SR11* (1997).

12. U.S. Department of Agriculture, Agricultural Research Service, "Composition of Foods: Raw, Processed, Prepared," *Agriculture Handbook No. 8* (1963).

13. U.S. Department of Agriculture, Agriculture Research Service, *Nutrient Database, SR11* (1997).

14. Hornick, S.B., "Factors affecting the nutritional quality of crops," *Am. J. Alt. Ag.* 7, nos.1 and 2 (1992).

15. Smith, B.L., "Organic foods vs. Supermarket foods: Element levels," *J. Appl. Nutr.* 45, no. 1 (1993): 35-38.

16. Langre, J.D., *Seasalt's Hidden Powers* (Happiness Press, 1994).

17. Kervran, C. Louis, *Biological Transmutations* (Magalia, CA: Happiness Press, 1988).

18. Laragh, John H., "Giving Salt a Fair Shake," *Health* (Cornell Hypertensive Center, 1986).

19. Bloch, G., "Dietary Guidelines and results of food consumption surveys," *Am. J. Clin. Nutr.* 53 (1979): 356-57.

20. Newnham, R.E., "Arthritis or Skeletal Fluorosis and Boron," *Int. Clin. Nutr. Rev.* 11 (1991): 68-70.

21. Guiness, A.D., ed., *The ABC's of the Human Body* (Pleasantville, NY: The Reader's Digest Assoc., Inc., 1987).

22. Hendler, S.S., *The Doctor's Vitamin and Mineral Encyclopedia* (New York: Simon & Schuster, 1990).

23. "Nutritive Value of American Foods in Common Units," *Agricultural Handbook,* USDA, No. 8-12 (1984).

24. Solomons, N.W., "Biochemical, metabolic, and clinical role in copper in human nutrition," *J. Am. Col. Nutr.* 4 (1985): 83-105.

25. Kivirikko, K., and Peltonen, L., "Abnormalities in copper metabolism and disturbances in the synthesis of collagen and elastin," *Med. Biol.* 60 (1982): 45-48.

26. Kameno, B., "Germanium: A New Approach to Immunity," *Nutrition Encounter* (1997).

27. Suzuki, F., and Pollard, R.B., "Prevention of Suppressed Interferon Gamma Production in Thermally Injured Mice by Administration of a Novel Organogermanium Compound, G-132," *Journal of Interferon Research* 4 (1984): 223-33.

28. Suzuki, F., et al., "Macrophage involvement in the protective effect of carboxyethylgermanium sesquioxide (GE-132) against nurine ascites tumors," *Int. J. Immunotherapy* 2 (1986): 239-45.

29. Satoh, H., and Iwaguchi, T., "Antitumor activity of new organogermanium compound. GE-132," *Gan to Kagaku Ryoko* 6 (1979): 79-83.

30. Jansson, B., "Dietary, Total Body, and Intracellular potassium-to-sodium ratios and their influence on cancer," *Cancer Detect. Prevent.* 14 (1991): 563-65.

31. National Research Council, *Diet and Health: Implications for Reducing Chronic Disease Risk* (Washington, DC: National Academy Press, 1989): 421-23.

32. Murray, F., *The Big Family Guide to All the Minerals* (New Cancer, CT: Keats Publishing, 1995).

33. Buffington, C.A.; Rogers, Q.R.; and Morris, J.G., "Feline Struvite urolithiasis: Magnesium effect depends on urinary pH," *Fel. Practice* 15 (1985): 29.

34. Torttelin, M.D., "Feline struvite urolithiasis: Factors affecting urine pH may be more important than magnesium levels in food," *Vet. Record* 121 (1987): 227.

35. Shanberger, R.J., et al., "Epidemiological studies on selenium and heart disease," *Fed. Proc.* 35 (1976): 578.

36. Wallach, J.D., and Lan, M., *Rare Earths: Forbidden Cures* (Bonita, CA: Double Happiness Publishing Co., 1994).

37. Shanberger, R.J., et al., "Epidemiological studies on selenium and heart disease," *Fed. Proc.* 35 (1976): 578.

38. Hocman, G., "Chemoprevention of Cancer: Selenium," *Int. J. Biochem.* 20 (1988): 123-32.

39. Kiremidijian-Schumacher, L., et al., "Supplementation with selenium and human immune cell function. Its effect on cytotoxic lymphocytes and natural killer cells," *Biological Trace Element Research* 41 (1994): 115-27.

40. Levander, O., and Beck, M., "Selenium deficiency results in viral virulence," *Journal of the Am. Col. of Nutr.* (1996).

41. Roy, M., "Supplementation with selenium and human immune cell functions; Effect on lymphocyte proliferation and Interleukin 2 receptor expression," *Biol. Trace Elem. Res.* 41 (1994): 103-14.

42. Tarp, U., et al., "Selenium Treatment in Rheumatoid Arthritis," *Scandinavian Journal of Rheumatology* (1985).

43. Bouvier, S., and Millart, H., "Relationship between selenium deficiency and 3, 5, 3 triiodothyronine (T3) synthesis," *Ann. Endocrinal* 58 (1997): 310-15.

44. Murray, F., *The Big Family Guide to All the Minerals* (New Caravan, CT: Keats Publishing, 1995).

45. MacDonald, A., *The Complete Book of Vitamins and Minerals* (Lincolnwood, IL: Publications International, 1996).

46. Herschuler, R.J., "Diet & Pharm Uses of MSM and Comp Comprising It," U.S. Patent 4, 513, 421 (April 3, 1985).

47. Jacobs, S.W., "The Current Status of MSM in Medicine," *Am. Acad. Med. Prev.* (1983).

48. Mindell, E.L., *The MSM Miracle* (New Caravan, CT: Keats Publishing, 1997).

49. Shils, M.E., and Young, U.R., *Modern Nutrition in Health and Disease* 7th ed. (Philadelphia: Delea and Kebiger, 1988).

50. Dardeme, M., et al., "Contribution of zinc and other metals to the biological activity of the serum thymic factor," *Proc. Natl. Acad. Sci.* 79 (1982): 5370-73.

51. Kunkle, G.A., "Zinc responsive dermatoses in dogs," in *Current Veterinary Therapy* 4 (1980) Kirk, R.W., ed.: 472-76.

CHAPTER 5

1. Pottinger, F., "The Effect of Heat Processed Foods and Metabolized Vitamin D Milk on the Dentofacial Structures of Experimental Animals," *Journal of Orthodontics and Oral Surgery* 32, no. 8 (August 1946): 467-85.

2. Price, W.A., *Nutrition and Physical Degeneration* (Price-Pottinger, Nutrition Foundation Publisher, 1982).

3. Howell, E., "Enzyme Starvation," *The Journal of the Am. Assoc. For Medico-Physical Research* (April 15, 1940).

4. Kantchakoff, P., "The Influence of Food on the Blood Formula of Man," First International Congress of Microbiology, Paris (1930).

5. Howell, E., *Enzyme Nutrition* (Avery Publishing, 1985).

6. Howell, E., *Food Enzymes for Health and Longevity* (Lotus Press, 1994).

7. Howell, E., *Enzyme Nutrition* (Avery Publishing, 1985).

8. Cichoke, A., *The Complete Book of Enzyme Therapy* (Avery Publishing, 1999).

9. Howell, E., *Enzyme Nutrition* (Avery Publishing, 1985).

10. Ibid.

11. Terrell, S.S., et al., "On Trial: An enzyme-producing food supplement for dogs," *Vet. Med.* 79, no. 11 (1984): 1367.

12. Knowles, R.P., and Basshon, H.H., "Clinical impressions of the use of an enzyme additive in large and small animals," *VM/SAC* 74, no. 12 (1979): 1733.

13. Cichoke, A., *Enzymes: Nature's Energizer* (Keats Publishing, Inc., 1997).

14. Wysong, R.L., *Rationale for Animal Nutrition* (Inquiry Press, 1998).

CHAPTER 6

1. *The Immune System—How it works*, National Institute of Health (Bethesda, MD: 1996).

2. Tizard, I., *Veterinary Immunology* 4th edition (W.B. Saunders, 1992).

3. Morra, M., and Potts, E., *Understanding Your Immune System* (New York: Avon Books, 1986).

4. Peakman, M., and Diego, V., *Basic and Clinical Immunology* (New York: Churchill Livingtone, 1997).

5. Herberman, R.B., and Gortaldo, J.R., "Natural Killer cells: Their role in defenses against disease," *Science* 214 (1981): 29-30.

6. Kelso, A., "TH_1 and TH_2 subsets: Paradigms lost?" *Immunol. Today* 16 (1995): 374-79.

7. Hnilica, K., and Angarano, D., "Role of T Helper Lymphocyte Subsets," *Comp. of Contin Ed.* (January 1997).

8. Modlin, R.L., "TH_1 and TH_2 paradigm: Insights from leprosy," *J. Invest. Dermatol.* 102 (1994): 828-31.

9. Brett, C., and Lafferty, K.J., "The TH_1/TH_2 balance in autoimmunity," *Curr. Opin. Immunol.* 7 (1985): 793-98.

10. Tizard, I., *Veterinary Immunology* 4th edition (W.B. Saunders, 1992).

11. Tyler, V.E., *Herbs of Choice: The Therapeutic Use of Phytomedicinals* (New York: Pharmaceutical Products Press, 1994).

12. Tsung, P.K., "Anticancer and immunostimulating polysaccharides," *OHAI Bulletin* 12 (1987): 1-10.

13. Dharmananda, S., "Medicinal Mushrooms," *Bestways Magazine* (July 1998).

14. Kohda, H., et al., "The Biologically Active Constituents of Ganoderma lucidum," *Chem. Pharm. Bull.* 33, no. 4 (1985): 1367-74.

15. Jiang, S., "Immunomodulating effects of cordyceps sinensis," *International Journal of Oriental Medicine* 16 (1991): 128-33.

16. Yan, S., et al., "Immune restoration and/or augmentation of local graft versus host reaction by traditional Chinese medicine herbs," *Cancer* 52 (1983): 70-73.

17. Yan, S., et al., "Effect of zholing polysaccharides on paritoneal macrophages on tumor- bearing mice," Proc. Int. Conf. on Trad. Chinese Med. and Pharm. (China Academic Publishers, 1988): 172-74.

18. Nio, Y., et al., "Immunomodulation by orally administered protein-bound polysaccharide PSK in patients with gastrointestinal cancer," *Biotherapy* 4, no. 2 (1992): 117-28.

19. Takai, M., et al., "Studies on the constituents of Astragali Radix," *Proc 25th Symposium of the Chemistry of Natural Products* 25 (Tokyo: 1982): 298-305.

20. Humphries, M.J., et al., *Cancer Research* 48 (1988): 1412-15.

21. Hov, Y., et al., "Effect of Radix Astragali on the Interferon System," *Chin. Med. J.* 94 (1981): 35- 40.

22. Yan, S., et al., "Immune restoration and/or augmentation of local graft versus host reaction by traditional Chinese medicine herbs," *Cancer* 52 (1983): 70-73.

23. DiLuzzio, N.R., "Immunopharmacology of glucan: a broad spectrum enhancer of host defense mechanisms," *Trends in Pharmacol.* 4 (1983): 344-47.

24. Di Luzio, N.R., et al., "Comparative tumor-inhibitory and antibacterial activity of soluble and particulate glucan," *N. J. Cancer* 24, no.6 (1979): 773-79.

25. Watson, D.L., et al., "Factors in ruminant colostrum that influences cell growth and murine IgE antibody responses," *Journal of Dairy Research* 59 (1992): 369-80.

26. Hurley, D.J., et al., "Evidence supporting the mechanism of enteric protection provided by colostrum whey led supplements," *Proc. of the Am. Assoc. Bovine Proc.* 27 (1995): 197-98.

27. Ogra, P., et al., "Colostrum derived immunity and maternal neonatal interaction," *Animals of New York Acad. of Ki.* 409 (1983): 82-92.

28. Janusz, M., and Lisowski, J., "Proline-rich polypeptide (PRP)—An immunomodulatory peptide from bovine colostrums," *Arch. Immuno. Ther. Exp.* 41 (1993): 275-79.

29. Nitsch, A., et al., "Clinical Use of Bovine Colostrum," *Journal of Orthomolecular Medicine* 13 (1998).

30. Halpern, G.M., *Cordyceps: China's Healing Mushroom* (New York: Avery Publishing Group, 1999).

31. Zong, Q., et al., "Pharmacological Action of the Polysaccharide from Cordyceps (Cordyceps sinensis)," *Zhongcaoyao* 16, no. 7 (1986): 306-11.

32. Kuang, Y.D., et al., "Studies of effects of Cordyceps sinensis on lymphocyte functions," *Shanghai Immunologic Journal* 9, no. 1 (1989): 6.

33. Cheng, Q.S., et al., "Regulatory effects on condyceps on cellular immunity in rats with chronic renal failure," *Nt. Med. J. China* 72, no. 1 (1992): 27.

34. Ren-He, X., et al., "Effects of Cordyceps sinensis on Natural Killer Activity and Colony Formation of B16 Melanoma," *Chinese Medical Journal* 105, no. 2 (1992): 97-101.

35. Zhong, M.Q., et al., "Polysaccharide Peptide (PSP) Restores Immunosuppresion Induced by Cyclophosphanide in Rats," *Am. Journal of Chinese Med.* XXU, no. 1 (1997): 27-35.

36. Torisu, M., et al., "Significant prolongation of disease free period gained by oral polysaccharide (PSK) administration after curative surgical operation of colerectal cancer," *Cancer Immunology Immunotherapy* 31, no. 5 (1990): 261-68.

37. Bone, Kerry, "Echinacea: What Makes it Work?" *Alternative Medicine Review* 2, no. 2 (1997), 87-93.

38. Bone, Kerry, Echinacea: When Should it be Used? *Alternative Medical Review* 2, no. 6 (1997): 451-58.

39. Parnham, M.J., "Benefit-risk assessment of the squeezed sap of the purple coneflower (Echinacea purpurea) for long-term oral immunstimulation," *Phytoneal.* 3, no. 1 (1996): 95-102.

40. Hobbs, C., *Ginseng: The Energy Herb* (Botanica Press, 1997).

41. Dharmananda, S., "Renshen Fenguangjian (Ginseng/Royal Jelly)," *Ohai Bulletin* (April 1998).

42. Jie, Y.H., et al., "Immunomodulatory effects of Panax ginseng C.A. Meyer in the mouse," *Agents and Actions* 15 (1984): 386-91.

43. Beutler, E., and Gelbart, T., "Plasma glutathione in health and in patients with malignant disease," *J. Lab. Clin. Med.* 105, no. 5 (1985): 581-84.

44. De Leve, L.D., and Kaplowitz, N., "Glutathione metabolism and its role in hepatotoxicity," *Pharmacal. Ther.* 52, no. 3 (1991): 287-305.

45. Julius, M., and Lang, C.A., et al., "Glutathione and morbidity in community-based sample of elderly," *J. Clin. Epidemial.* 47, no. 9 (1994): 1021-26.

46. Jenner, P., "Altered mitochondrial function, iron metabolism and glutathione levels in Parkinson's disease," *Acts Neural. Scand. Suppl.* 146 (1993): 6-13.

47. Noelle, R.J., and Lawrence D.A., "Determination of glutathione in lymphocytes and possible association of redox state and proliferative capacity of lymphocytes," *Biochem. J.* 198 (1981): 571-79.

48. Newberne, P.M., and Butler, W.A., "Acute and chronic effects of aflatoxins B[1] on the liver of domestic and laboratory animals: a review," *Cancer Res.* 29 (1969): 236-50.

49. Peterson, J.D., et al., "Glutathione levels in antigen presenting cells modulate TH[1] versus TH[2] response patterns," *Proc. Natl. Acad. Sci. USA* 95 (1998): 3071-76.

50. Ohlenschager, G., and Treusch, G., "Reduced Glutathione and anthocyanins: Redox cycling and redox recycling in living systems," *Praxis-Telegramm* no. 6 (1994): 1-20.

51. Hagan, T.M., et al., "Bioavailability of dietary glutathione: effect on concentration," *Am. J. Physiol.* 259, no. 4 (1990): 524-29.

52. Hagan, T.M., et al., "Glutathione uptake and protection against oxidative injury in isolated kidney cells," *Kidney Ins.* 34, no. 1 (1988): 74-81.

53. Witschi, A., et al., "Supplementation of N-acetylcysteine Fails to Increase Glutathione in Lymphocytes and Plasma of Patients with AIDS," *Res. Hum. Retroviruses* no.11 (1995): 141-43.

54. Hauer, J., and Anderer, F.A., "Mechanism of stimulation of human natural killer cytotoxicity by arabinogalactan from Larix accidentalis," *Cancer Immunology Immunotherapy* 36 (1993): 237-44.

55. Ibid.

56. Vine, A.J., et al., "The effect of lactulose, pectin, arabinogalactan, and cellulose on the production of organic acids and metabolism of ammonia by intestinal bacteria in a fecal incubation system," *BL. J. Nutr.* 63 (1990): 17-26.

57. Hagmar, B., Ryd, W., and Shomedal, H., "Arabinogalactan blockade of experimental metastasis to liver by murine hepatoma," *Invasion Metastasis* 11 (1991): 348-55.

58. Nanba, H., "Maitake mushroom: Immune therapy to prevent from cancer growth and metastasis," *Explore* 6, no. 1 (1995).

59. Nanba, H., "Activity of Maitake D-Fraction to inhibit Carcinogensis and Metastasis," *Cancer Prevention* 768 (1995): 243-45.

60. Nanba, H., "Maitake mushroom: Immune therapy to prevent from cancer growth and metastasis," *Explore* 6, no. 1 (1995).

61. Hobbs, C., *Medicinal Mushrooms: An Exploration of Tradition, Healing and Culture* (Botanica Press, 1995).

62. Flynn, M.S., and Roest, M., *Guide to Standardized Herbal Products* (One World Press, 1995).

63. Lee, W.H., and Friedrich, J.A., *Medicinal Benefits of Mushrooms* (Keats Publishing, Inc., 1997).

64. Morishige, F., et al., "The Role of Vitamin C in Tumor Therapy" in *Vitamins and Cancer Prevention by Vitamins and Micronutrients*, Meyskena, F.L., and Prasad, K.N., eds. (Humana Press, 1986): 399-427.

65. Kupin, V.A., "New Biological Response Modifer-Ganoderma lucidurm—and its application in oncology," 4th International Symposium on Ganoderma Lucidum (June 10, 1992).

66. Chang, M.H., ed. Lingzhi, in *Pharmacology and Applications of Chinese Materica Medica* (Singapore: World Scientific, 1986).

67. Lee, W.H., and Friedrich, J.A., *Medicinal Benefits of Mushrooms* (Keats Publishing, Inc., 1997).

68. Aoki, T., "Lentinan: Immunemodulating Agents and Their Mechanisms," *Immunology Studies* 25 (1984): 62-77.

69. Tani, M., et al., "In vitro generation of activated natural killer cells and cytoxic macrophages with lentinan," *Eur. J. Clin. Pharmacol.* 42 (1992): 623-27.

70. Arinaga, S., et al., "Enhanced production of interleukin-1 and tumor necrosis factor by peripheral monocytes after lentinan administration in patients with gastric carcinoma," *Int. J. Immunopharmacol.* 14 (1992): 43-47.

71. Bouic, P.J.D., and Lamprecht, J., "Plant Sterols and Sterolins: A Review of Their Immunemodulating Properties," *Alt. Med. Rev.* 4, no. 3 (1999).

72. Gupta, M.B., et al., "Anti-inflammatory and anti-pyretic activities of b-sitosterol," *Plants Med* 39 (1980): 157-63.

73. Bouic, P.J.D., and Lamprecht, J., "Plant Sterols and Sterolins: A Review of Their Immunemodulating Properties," *Alt. Med. Rev.* 4, no. 3 (1999).

74. Bouic, P.J.D., "Immunomodulation in HIV/AIDS: The Tygerberg-Stellenbasch University experience," *AIDS Bulletin* 6, no. 3 (Medical Research Council of South Africa, 1997): 18-20.

75. Bouic, P.J.D., et al., "The effects of B-sitosteal (855) and B-sitosteral glycoside (BSSG) mixture on selected immune parameters of marathon runners: inhibition of post marathon immune suppression and inflammation," *Int. J. Sports Med.* (1999).

76. Bouic, P.J.D., "Sterols/Sterolins: The natural, nontoxic immunomodulators and their role in the control of rheumatoid arthritis," *The Arthritis Trust Newsletter* (1998).

77. Murray, M., *Glandular Extracts. What you must know. How natural concentrates stimulate endocrines, provide enzymes and promote cellular repair* (New Canaan, CT: Keats Publishing, 1994).

78. Cazzola, P., et al., "In vivo modulating effect of a calf thymus acid lusate on human T lymphocyte subsets and CD4+/CD8+ ratio in the causes of different diseases," *Cur. Ther. Res.* 42 (1987): 1011-17.

79. Kouttab, N.M., Proda, M., and Cazzola, P., "Thymomodulin: Biological properties and clinical applications," *Medical Oncology and Tumor Pharmacotherapy* 6 (1989): 5-9.

80. Fiocchi, A., et al., "A double-blind clinical trial for the evaluation of the therapeutic effectiveness of a calf thymus derivative (thymomodalin) in children with recurrent respiratory infections," *Thymus* 8 (1986): 831-39.

81. Cazzola, P., et al., "In vivo modulating effect of a calf thymus acid lusate on human T lymphocyte subsets and CD4+/CD8+ ratio in the causes of different diseases," *Cur. Ther. Res.* 42 (1987): 1011-17.

82. Marzari R., et al., "Perennial allergic rhinitis: Prevention of the acute episodes with thymomodulin," *Min. Med.* 78 (1987): 1675-81.

83. Genova, R., and Guerra, A., "Thymomodulin in management of food allergy in children," *Int. J. Tiss. React.* 8 (1986): 239-92.

84. Schauss, A.G., "Cat's Claw (uncaria tomentosa)" *Natural Medicine Journal* 1, no. 2 (March 1998).

85. Aquino, R., et al., "Plant metabolites. New compounds and anti-inflammatory activity of uncaria tomentosa," *J. of Nat. Products* 54 (1991): 453-59.

86. Keplinger, K., et al., "Uncaria tomentosa (WILD)DC. Ethnomedicinal use and new pharmacological, toxicological and botanical results," *J. Ethnopharmacol.* 64 (1999): 23-24.

87. Wurm, M., et al., "Pentacyclic oxindole alkaloids from uncaria tomentosa induce human endothelial cells to release a lymphocyte proliferation-regulating factor," *Plants Medica* 64 (1998): 701-4.

88. Stuppner, H., et al., "A Differential Sensitivity of Oxindole Alkaloids to Normal and Leukemic Cell Liver," *Planta Medica* 59, Suppl. (1993).

CHAPTER 7

1. Schwassmann, M., "Demodicous in Dogs," *Veterinary Forum* (July 1997): 42-45.

2. Scott, D.W., Miller, W.H., and Griffin, C.E., *Small Animal Dermatology*, 5th ed. (Philadelphia: W.B. Saunders, 1995).

3. Ristic, Z., et al., "Ivermectin for treatment of generalized demodicosis in dogs," *J. Am. Vet. Med. Assoc.* 10 (1995): 1308-10.

4. DeBoer, D.J., et al., "Evaluation of a commercial staphylococcal bacteria for management of idiopathic recurrent superficial pyoderma in dogs," *Am. J. Vet. Res.* 51, no. 4 (1990): 636-39.

5. Nesbit, G.H., and Ackerman, L.J., "Dermatology for the small animal practitioner," *Vet. Learning Systems* (1991).

6. Saarinen, U.M., and Kajoseari, M., "Breast-feeding as prophylaxis against atopic disease: Propective follow-up study until 17 years old," *Lancet* 346 (1995): 1065-69.

7. Soter, N., and Boden, H., *Pathophysiology of Dermtalogic Disease* (New York: McGraw-Hill, 1984).

8. Liechtenstein, L.M., "Allergy and the immune system," *Scientific America* (September 1993): 116-24.

9. Vanderhaeghe, L.R., and Bouic, P.J.D., *The Immune System Cure: Nature's Way to Super-Powered Health* (Prentice Hall, 1999).

10. Muller, G.H., et al., *Cutaneous Endocrinology: Small Animal Dermatology*, 4th ed. (Philadelphia: W.B. Saunders, 1989).

11. Reedy, L.M., Miller, W.H., and Willense, T., *Allergic Skin Diseases of Dogs and Cats* (W.B. Saunders, 1997).

12. Nakagawa, T., "The role of IgG subclass antibodies in the clinical response to immunotherapy in allergic disease," *Clin. Exp. Allergy* 21 (1991): 289-96.

13. Nish, W.A., et al., "The effect of immunotherapy on the cutaneous late phase response to antigen," *J. Allergy Clin. Immunol.* 93, no. 2 (1994): 484-94.

14. White, S.D., "Food Allergy in Dogs," *Comp. Cont. Ed.* 20, no. 3 (March 1998).

15. Miller, S.B., "IgG Food Allergy Testing by Elisa/EIA: What do They Really Tell Us," *Townsend Letter for Doctors and Patients* (January 1998).

16. Weiner, M.A., and Weiner, J.A., *Herbs That Heal: Prescription for Herbal Healing.* (Quantum Books, 1994).

17. Ammon, H.P., and Wahl, M.A., "Pharmacology of Curcuma longa," *Planta Medica* 57, no.1 (1991): 1- 7.

18. Ammon, H.P., and Safayhi, H., et al., "Mechanism of anti-inflammatory actions of curcumin and boswellic acids," *J. Ethnopharmacal.* 38 (1993): 117-19.

19. Makheja, A.M., et al., "A platelet phospholipase inhibitor from the medicinal herb feverfew (tanacetum parthenium)," *Prostogland. Leukotri. Med.* 8 (1982): 653-60.

20. Murray, M.T., and Buetlar, J., *Understanding Fats and Oils: Your Guide to Healing with Essential Fatty Acids* (Progressive Health Publishing, 1996).

21. Shukla, V.K., et al., "The presence of oxidative polymeric materials in encapsulated fish oils," *Lipids* 26 (1991): 1.

22. Cho, Sung-Hee, and Choi, Young-son, "Lipid peroxidation and antioxidant status is affected by different vitamin E levels when feeding fish oil," *Lipids* 29, no. 1 (1994).

23. Brown, D.J., *Herbal Prescription for Better Health* (Prima Publishing, 1996).

24. Kuchi, F., and Iwakami, S., et al., "Inhibition of prostaglandin and leukotriene biosynthesis by gingerols and dioylheptanoids," *Chem. Pharm. Bull.* 40 (1992): 387-91.

25. Roundtree, R., "Licorice and corticosteroids: Double-edged swords," *Herbs for Health* (March/April 2000).

26. Della, L., et al., "Anti-inflammatory activity of benzopyrones that are inhibitors of cyclo- and lipo-oxygenase," *Pharmacol. Res. Commun.* 20 (1988): 591-94.

27. Kim, H.P., et al., "Effects of naturally occurring flavonoids and bioflavonoids on epidermal cycloxygenase from guinea pigs," *Prostaglandins Leakot. Essent. Fatty Acids* 58 (1998): 17-24.

28. Bronner, C., and Landy, Y., "Kinetics of the inhibitory effects of flavonoids on histamine secretion from most cells," *Agents Actions* 16 (1985): 147-56.

29. Castillo, M.H., et al., "The effects of the bioflavonoid quercitin or squamous cell carcinoma of head and neck origin," *Am. J. Suppl.* 158 (1989): 351-55.

CHAPTER 8

1. Murray, M.T., *Arthritis: How You Can Benefit from Diet, Vitamins, Minerals, Herbs, Exercise and Other Natural Methods* (Ricklin, CA: Prima Publishing, 1994).

2. Timm, Arne, *Influence of Gelatin Feed on the Skeletal System, Hair, Cartilage and Hoof Horn Growth of Yearling Foals* (Hanover, 1993).

3. Seeligmuller, K., and Happez, H.K., "Can a mixture of gelatin and L-cystine stimulate protroglycan synthesis," *Therapiewoche* 39 (1989): 3153-57.

4. Goetz, B., "Chrondropathia Patellae," *Aerzliche Praxis.* 92 (1982): 3130-34.

5. Adam, M., "Osteoarthrosis therapy in gelatin preparations: results of clinical study," *Therapiewoche* 38 (1991): 2456-61.

6. Murray, M.T., "Irrefutable evidence: Glucosamine sulfate proven superior over other forms of glucosamine and chondroitin sulfate" (Vital Communications, Inc.)

7. Murray, M.T., "Glucasanine sulfate vs. other forms of glucosamine and chondroitin sulfates," *Am. Journal of Nat. Med.* (1997).

8. Gibson, R.G., et al., "The anti-inflammatory activity of perna canaliculus," *New Zealand Medical Journal* 92 (1980): 667.

9. Dharmananda, S., "Sea Cucumber," Institute for Traditional Medicine, Portland, OR (April 1998).

CHAPTER 9

1. Cotter, S.M., "Oral pharyngeal neoplasms in the cats," *J. Am. Anim. Hosp. Assoc.* 17 (1981): 917.

2. Liehr, H., and Grun, M., *Progress in Liver Disease* (New York: Grune and Straten, 1979): 313-26.

3. Thenev, N., "The Scientific Criteria For Selecting Efficacious Probiotics," *Townsend Letter for Doctors* (November 1994).

4. Gittleman, A.L., *Beyond Probiotics: The Revolutionary Rediscovery of a Missing Link in Our Immune System* (New Canaan, CT: Keats Publishing, Inc., 1998).

5. Zimmes, J.F., and Burrington, D.B., "Comparison of Four Protocols for Treatment of Canine Giardiasis," *JAAHA* 22 (1986): 168-72.

6. Grove, D.I., et al., "Suppression of cell-mediated immunity of netronidazole," *Int. Arch. Allergy Appl. Immunol.* 5 (1977): 422-27.

7. Miller, A.L., "The Pathogenesis, Clinical Implications and Treatment of Intestinal Hyperpermeability," *Alt. Med. Rev.* 2, no. 5 (1997): 330-45.

8. Miller, A.L., "Therapeutic Considerations of L-Glutamine: A review of the literature," *Alt. Med. Rev.* 4, no. 4 (1999): 239-48.

9. Ward, P.D., and Young, G.P., "Dynamics of Clostridium difficile infection. Control using diet," *Adv. Exp. Med. Biol.* 412 (1997): 63-75.

10. Otamiri, T., and Tagesson, C., "Ginkgo bilba extract prevents mucosal damage associated with small-intestinal ischemia," *Scand. J. Gest.* 24 (1989): 666-70.

11. Campbell, J.M., et al., "Selected indigestible aligosaccharides affect large bowel mass, cecal and fecal short-chain fatty acids, pH and microflora in rats," *J. Nutr.* 127 (1997): 130-36.

12. Hills, J.M., and Aaronson, P.I., "The Mechanism of Action of Peppermint Oil in Gastrointestinal Smooth Muscle," *Gastroent.* 101 (1991): 55-65.

13. McKinnon, R.A., and Nebert, D.W., "Possible role of cytochrome P-450 in lupus erythematosis and related disorders," *Lupus* 3 (1994): 473-78.

14. Liska, D.J., "The Detoxification Enzyme Systems," *Alt. Med. Rev.* 2, no. 3 (1998): 187-98.

15. Adzet, T., et al., "Hepatoprotective activity of polyphenolic compounds from cynara scalymnus against cc/4 toxicity in isolated rat hepatocytes," *J. Nat. Prod.* 50 (1987): 612.

16. Ibid.

17. Pizzorno, J., *Total Wellness: Improve Your Health by Understanding the Body's Healing Systems* (Prima Publishing, 1996).

18. Kendall, R.V., and Lawson, J.W., "Recent Findings on N, N-Dimethylglycine (DMG): A Nutrient for the New Millennium," *Townsend Letter for Doctors and Patients* (May 2000).

19. Graber, G., and Kendall, R., "N, N-Dimethyglycine and use in immune response," US Patient, 4,631, 189 (December 1986).

20. Slaga, T.J., and Quilici-Timmcke, J., *D-Glucarate: A Nutrient Against Cancer* (Los Angeles: Keats Publishing, 1999).

21 Dutton, G.J., *Glucuronidation of Drugs and Other Compounds* (Boca Raton, FL: CRC Press, 1980).

22. Luper, S., "A Review of Plants Used in the Treatment of Liver Disease: Part two," *Alt. Med. Rev.* 4, no. 3 (1999): 178-88.

23. Kiso, Y., et al., "Mechanism of antihepatotoxic activity of glycyrrhizin: effect on free radical generation and lipid peroxidation," *Planta Medica* 50 (1984): 298-302.

24. Moon, A., and Kim, S.H., "Effect of Glycyrrhiza glabra roots and glycyrrhizin on the glucurronidation in rats," *Planta Medica* 63 (1997): 115-19.

25. Fujisawa, K., et al., "Therapeutic effects of liver hydrolysate preparation on chronic hepatitis—a double-blind, controlled study," *Asian Med. J.* 26 (1984): 497-526.

26. Tuchweber, B., et al., "Prevention by silibinin of phalloidin induced hepatotoxicty," *Toxicol. Appl. Pharm.* 51 (1979): 265-75.

27. Valenzuela, A., et al. "Selectivity of silymarin on the increase of the glutathione content in different tissues of the rat," *Planta Medica* 55 (1989): 42.

28. Sonnenbichler, J., et al., "Stimulation effects of silibinin on the DNA-synthesis in partially hepatectomized rat livers: non-response in hepatoma and other malignant cell lines," *Biochem. Pharm.* 35 (1986): 538-41.

29. Halim, A.B., et al, "Biochemical effects of antioxidants on lipids and liver function in experimentally induced liver damage," *Am. Clin. Bioch.* 34 (1997): 656-63.

30. Ferenci, R., et al, "Randomized controlled trial of silymarin treatment in patients with cirrhosis of the liver," *J. Hepatology* 9 (1989): 105-13.

31. Bone, K., "Picrorhiza: important modulator of immune friction," *Townsend Letter for Doctors* (May 1995).

32. Chandeler, R., et al., "Effect of picroliv on glutathione metabolism in liver and brain of mastomys matalensis infected with plasmodium bergha," *Indian J. Exp. Biol.* 30 (1992): 711-14.

33. Singh, V., et al., "Effect of picroliv on protein and nucleic acid synthesis," *Indian J. Exp. Biol.* 30 (1992): 68-69.

34. Stolk, J., et al., "Characteristics of the inhibition of NaDPH oxidase activation in neutrophils by apocynin, a methoxy-substituted catechol," *Am. J. Respir. Cell Mol. Biol.* 11 (1994): 95-102.

35. Luper, S., "A review of plants used in the treatment of liver disease: Part 1," *Alt. Med. Rev.* 3, no. 6 (1998): 410-21.

36. Santra, A., et al., "Prevention of carbon tetrachloride-induced hepatic injury in mice by picrorhiza kurroa," *Indian J. Gastroenterol.* 17 (1998): 6-9.

37. Shukla, B., Visen, P.K., and Patnaik, G.K., "Choleretic effect of picroliv, the hepatoprotective principle of picrorhiza kurroa," *Planta Medica* 57 (1991): 329-33.

38. *Disease Prevention and Treatment* 3rd edition (Life Extension Foundation, 2000): 405-406.

39. Gaeddert, A., "What is SAM? Ask the Herbalist," *Townsend Letter for Doctors* (June 2000).

40. Angelico, M., "Oral S-adenosylmethionine (SAM) administration enhancing bile salt conjugation with taurine in patients with liver cirrhosis," *Scand. J. Clin. Lab. Invest.* 54 (1994): 459-64.

41. Osman, E., et al., "Review article: S- adenosylmethionine—a new therapeutic agent in liver disease?" *Aliment Pharmacol. Ther.* 7, no. 1 (1993): 21-28.

CHAPTER 10

1. Horrobin, D.R., "Review article: Medical uses of essential fatty acids (EFAs)," *Vet. Dermatol.* 4 (1993): 161-66.

2. Anderson, J.W., et al., "Effects of psyllium on glucose and serum lipid responses in men with Type II diabetes and hypercholesterolemia," *Am. J. Clin. Nutr.* 70 (1999): 466-73.

3. Carreau, J.P., "Biosynthesis of lipoic acid via unsaturated fatty acids," *Methods Enzymol.* 62 (1979): 152-58.

4. Heller, B., and Burkhart, V., et al., "Antioxidant therapy for the prevention of Type I diabetes," *Adv. Pharm.* 38 (1997): 629-38.

5. Estrada, E.E., et al., "Stimulation of glucose uptake by the natural coenzyme alpha-lipoic acid/thioctic acid: participation of elements of the insulin signaling pathway," *Diabetes* 45 (1996): 1798-1804.

6. Jacobs, S., and Russ, P., et al., "Oral administration of rac-a-lipoic acid modulates insulin sensitivity in patients with Type II diabetes mellitus in a placebo-controlled pilot trial," *Free Raic. Biol. Med.* 27 (1999): 309-14.

7. Anderson, C.B., et al., "The effect of coenzyme Q_{10} on blood glucose and insulin requirement in patients with insulin-dependent diabetes mellitus," *Molec. Aspects Med.* 18 (1997): 307-309.

8. McCarty, M.D., "Can correction of sub-optimal coenzyme Q status improve beta cell function in Type II diabetics?" *NutriGuard Research* 52, no. 5 (May 1999): 397-400.

9. Jacobs, B.M., *Coenzyme Q_{10}: All-around Nutrient for All-around Health* (Temecula, CA: BL Publications, 1999).

10. Marles, N.R., "Antidiabetic plants and their active constituents," *Protocol Journal of Botanical Medicine* (Winter 1996).

11. Bies, G., et al., "Antidiabetic effect of subfractions from fenugreek seeds in diabetic dogs," *Proc. Sec. Exp. Biol. Med.* 182, no. 2 (1986): 159-66.

12. Varma, D., "Inhibition of aldose reductase by flavonoids: possible attenuation of diabetic complications," *Prog. Clin. Biol. Res.* 213 (1986): 343-58.

13. DeCava, J.A., "The Chromium Controversy," *Nutrition News and Views* 2, no. 2 (March/April 1998): 1.

14. Prakash, A.O., et al., "Effect of feeding gymnema sylvestre leaves on blood glucose in beryllium nitrate treated rats," *J. Ethnopharmacol.* 18 (1986): 143-46.

15. Shanmugasundaram, E.R., et al., "Possible regeneration of the islets of langerhans in streptozotocin—diabetic rats given gymnema sylvestre leaf extracts," *J. Ethnopharmacol.* 302 (1996): 265-79.

16. Shanmugasundaram, E.R., et al., "Use of gymnema sylvestre leaf in the control of blood glucose in insulin-dependent diabetes melltisu," *J. Ethnopharmacol.* 30 (1990): 281-94.

17. Cunnick, J., and Takeomto, D., "Bitter Melon (Mormordica charantia)," *J. Nat. Med.* 4 (1993): 16- 21.

18. Baldwa, C.M., et al., "Clinical Trials in Patients with Diabetes Mellitus of an insulin-like compound obtained from plant sources," *Lipoala J. Med. Sci.* 82 (1977): 39-41.

19. Khanna, P., et al., "Hypoglycemic activity of polypeptide-p from a plant source," *J. Nat. Prod.* 44 (1981): 648-55.

20. Cignarella, A., et al., "Novel lipid-lowering properties of vaccinium myrtillus L. leaves, a traditional antidiabetic treatment in several models of rat dyslipidemia: a comparison with ciprofibrate," *Thromb. Res.* 84 (1996): 311-22.

21. Boniface, R., and Robert, A.M., "Effect of anthocyanins on human connective tissue metabolism in the human in Monatable augenheilkd," 209 (1996): 368-72.

22. Mooradian, A.D., and Morley, J.E., "Micronutrient status in diabetes mellitus," *J. Clin. Nutr.* 45 (1987): 877-95.

23. Hegazi, S.M., et al., "Effect of zinc supplementation on serum supplementation glucose- 6-phosphatase, and mineral levels in diabetes," *J. Clin. Biochem. Nutr.* 12 (1992): 209-215.

24. Nichols, R., et al., "Hypoadrenocorticisn," in Birchard, S.J., and Sheriding, R.G., (eds): *Saunders Manual of Small Animal Practice* (Philadelphia: W.G. Saunders Co., 1994): 238-40.

25. Kelch, W.J., et al., "Canine hypoadrenocorticism (Addison's Disease)," *Compendium on Cont. Ed.* 20, no. 8 (1998): 921-34.

26. Ferguson, D., et al., *Endocrinologic Disorders in Small Animal Medical Therapeutics* (Ed) Lorenz, M.D., Cornelius, L.M., and Ferguson, D.C. (Philadelphia: J.B. Lippincott Co., 1992).

27. Ibid.

28. DeCava, J.A., "Underactive and Overactive Thyroid," *Nutrition News and Views* 3, no. 4 (1999).

29. Ibid.

30. Peterson, M.E., "Measurement of serum total thyroxine, triiodthyronine, free thyroxine, and thyrotropin concentrations for diagnosis of hypothyroidism in dogs," *J.A.V.M.A.* 211, no. 11 (1997): 1396-1402.

31. Dodds, J.W., "Canine autoimmune thyroiditis: 1,000 cases," in proceedings of A.H.V.M.A. (1999).

32. Valentine, T., "If you Eat Soy, Watch Your Thyroid Function, New Study," *Time Health Quarterly Newsletter* (Autumn 1997).

33. Toto, T., "Selenium's role in thyroid found," *New Scientist* 129 (1991).

34. Berry, M.J., and Larsen, P.R., "The role of selenium in thyroid hormone action," *Endocrine Review* 13 (1992): 207-20.

CHAPTER 11

1. Avorn, J., et al., "Reduction of bacteriuria and pyuria after ingestion of cranberry juice," *JAMA* 271, no. 10 (1994): 751-54.

2. Howell, A.B., Vora, N., Der Mardersonian, A., and Foo, L.Y., "Inhibition of the adherence of p-finbriated Escherichia coli to ureopithelial-cell surfaces by proanthocyanidin extracts from cranberries," *N. Eng. J. Med.* 339, no. 15 (1998): 1085-86.

3. Zafriri, D., et al., "Inhibitory activity of cranberry juice on adherence of type-1 and type-p fimbriated escherichia coli to eucaryotic cells," *Antimicrobial Agents and Chemotherapy* 33, no. 1 (1989): 72-98.

4. Ofek, I., et al., "Anti-Escherichia Activity of Cranberry and Blueberry Juices," *N. Eng J. Med.* 324 (1991): 1597-1791.

5. Weiss, R.F., *Herbal Medicine* (A.B. Arcanum, Gothenburg: Beaconsfield Publishers, 1988).

6. Larson, B., et al., "Prophylactic effect of UVA-E in Women with Recurrent Cystitis: A Preliminary Report," *Curr. Ther. Res.* 53 (1993): 441-43.

7. Kruber, J.M., Osborne, C.A., and Goyal, S.M., et al., "Clinical evaluation of cats with lower urinary tract disease," *JAVMA* 199 (1991): 211-16.

8. Buffington, C.A.T., et al., "Clinical evaluation of cats with nonobstructive urinary tract diseases," *JAVMA* 210 (1997): 46-50.

9. Osborne, C.A., et al., "Feline lower urinary tract disease: The Minnesota experience," *Proc. 15th Acutim Forum* (1997): 328-39.

10. Kruber, J.M., Osborne, C.A., and Goyal, S.M., et al., "Clinical evaluation of cats with lower urinary tract disease," *JAVMA* 199 (1991): 211-16.

11. Senior, D.F., and Brown, M.D., "The role of Mycroplasma species and Ureaplasma species in feline lower urinary tract disease," *Vet. Clin. North Am.* 26, no. 2 (1996): 305-308.

12. Martens, J.G., et al., "The role of infectious agents in naturally occurring feline urological syndrome," *Vet. Clin. North Am.* 14 (1984): 503-11.

13. Kalkstein, T.S., Kruger, J.M., and Osborne, C.A., "Feline Idiopathic Lower Urinary Tract Disease. Part II: Potential Causes," *Comp. Cont. Ed.* 21, no. 2 (1999): 148-54.

14. Buffington, C.A.T., et al., "Interstitial cystitis in cats," *Vet. Clin. North Am.* 26 (1996): 317-26.

15. Robertson, J.L., "Immunologic injury to the kidney and the renal response" in Bovee, K.C., (ed): *Canine Nephrology* (Media, PA: Harvard Publishing Co., 1984): 439-60.

16. Hosford, A., et al., "Natural Antagonists of platelet-activating factor phytotherapy," *Research* 2, no.1 (1988): 1-25.

17. Grino, T., "BN 52021: A Platelet Activating Factor Antagonist for Preventing Post-Transplant Renal Failure—A Double-Blind, Randomized Study," *Ann. Intern. Med.* 121 (1994): 345-47.

18. Sugano, M., et al., "A novel use of chitosan as a hypocholesterolemic agent in rats," *Ann. J. of Clin. Nutr.* 33, no. 4 (1980): 787-73.

19. Halpern, G., *Cordyceps: China's Healing Mushroom* (Avery Publishing Group, 1999).

20. Tian, J., et al., "Effects of Cordyceps sinensis, Rhubarb and Serum Renatrpin on Tubular Epitherlial Cell Growth," *Chung Hsi Chieh Ho Tsa Chih* 11, no. 9 (1991): 518, 547-49.

21. Li, L., et al., "Clinical Protection of Aminoglycoside Nephrotoxcity by Cordyceps sinensis," *J. of the Am. Soc. of Neph.* 3, no. 3 (1992): 726.

22. Jiang, J.C., and Cao, Y.F., "Summary of Treatment of 37 Chronic Renal Dysfunction Patients with Jin Shaibao," *J. of Admin. of Trad. Chi. Med.* 5 (1995): 23-24.

23. Hamm, L.L., et al., "Epidermal Growth Factor and the Kidney," *Seminars in Nephrology* 13, no. 1 (1993): 109-15.

24. Takako, Y., et al., "Increase of Active Oxygen in Rats after Nephrectomy Is Suppressed by Ginsing Sopinin," *Phytotherapy Research* 10 (1996): 569-72.

25. Tomoda, M., et al., "Structural features and anticomplementary activity of rehmannan SA, a polysaccharide from the root of rehamannia glutinosa," *Chem. Pharm. Bull.* 42, no. 8 (1994): 1666-68.

26. Takako, Y., et al., "Effects of Rhubarb Extract in Rats in Diabetic Nephropathy," *Phytotherapy Research* 11 (1997): 73-75.

27. Hua, Gao, and Lien, Eric, "Chemistry and Pharmacology of Salvia miltiorrhiza Radix," *Int. J. of Orient. Med.* 17, no. 3 (1992): 125-33.

28. Takako, Y., et al., "Renal Responses to Magnesium Lithospermate B(MLB) in Rats with Adenine-Induced Renal Failure," *Phyt. Res.* 7 (1993): 235-39.

29. Ye, G., et al., "Effects of Polipsaccharides Purified from Salvia miltiorrhiza radix on experimental nephrosis in rats," *Phyt. Res.* 8 (1994): 237-341.

30. Lohmann, A., et al., "Investigation of the Possible Influence of Vinpocetine with Concomitant Application of Magnesium-alluminun-hydroxide GEL," *Argneim-Forsch/Drug Res.* 41, no. 2 (1991): 1164-67.

31. Newburgh, L.H., and Curtis, A.C., "Production of renal injury in the white rat by the protein of the diet," *Arch. Int. Med.* 42 (1928): 801-21.

32. Addis, T., et al., "The relation between the serum urea concentration and the protein consumption of normal individuals," *J. Clin. Invest.* 26 (1947): 869-74.

33. *Nutritional Requirements of Dogs* (Washington, DC: National Research Council, National Academy of Science, 1972).

34. Bovee, K.C., and Kronfeld, D.S., "Reduction of Renal hemodynamics in uremic dogs fed reduced protein diets," *JAAHA* 17 (1981): 277.

35. Polzin, D.J., et al., "Influence of modified protein diets on the nutritional status of dogs with induced chronic renal failure," *Am. J. Vet. Res.* 44 (1983): 1694-1702.

36. Polzin, D.J., et al., "Influence of reduced protein diets on morbidity, mortality and renal function in dogs with induced chronic renal failure," *Am. J. Vet. Res.* 45 (1984): 506-17.

37. Polzin, D.J., et al., "Development of renal lesions in dogs after 11/12 reduction of renal mass: influences of dietary protein intake," *Lab. Invest.* 58 (1988): 172-83.

38. White, J.V., et al., "Effect of dietary protein on functional, morphologic and histologic changes of the kidney during compensatory renal growth in dogs," *Am. J. Vet. Res.* 52 (1991): 1357-65.

39. Finco, D.R., and Brown, S.A., et al., "Effects of aging and dietary protein intake on uninephrectomized geriatric dogs," *Am. J. Vet. Res.* 55 (1994): 1282-90.

CHAPTER 12

1. DeCava, J.A., "Congestive Heart Failure," *Nutrition News and Views* 1, no. 5 (1997).

2. Sinatra, S.T., *Coenzyme Q_{10} and the Heart* (Los Angeles: Keats Publishing, 1997).

3. Jacobs, B.M.L., *Coenzyme Q10: All-Around Nutrient for All-Around Health* (Temecula, CA: BL Publishing, 1999).

4. Baggio, E., et al., "Italian multicenter study on the safety and efficacy of coenzyme Q_{10} as adjunctive therapy in heart failure, CoQ_{10} Drug Surveillance investigators," *Mol. Aspects Med.* 15 (1994): 287-94.

5. Langsjoen, H., et al., "Usefulness of coenzyme Q_{10} in clinical cardiology: A long-term study," *Mol. Aspects Med.* 15 (1994): 165-75.

6. Morisco, C., et al., "Effect of coenzyme Q_{10} therapy in patients with congestive heart failure: a long-term multicenter randomized study," *Clin. Invest.* 71 (1993): 134-36.

7. Langsjoen, H., et al., "Pronounced increase of survival of patients with cardiomyopathy when treated with coenzyme Q_{10} and conventional therapy," *Int. J. Tissue React.* 12, no. 3 (1990): 163-68.

8. Yamagami, T., et al., "Bioenergetics in clinical medicine. Administration of coenzyme Q_{10} to patients with essential hypertension," *Res. Commun. Chem. Pathal. Pharmalol.* 14, no. 4 (1976): 721-27.

9. Langsjoen, H., "Effective and safe therapy with coenzyme Q_{10} for cardiomyopathy," *Klin Wocheuschi* 66, no. 13 (1988): 583-89.

10. Oda,T., "Recovery of load-induced left ventricular diastolic dysfunction by coenzyme Q_{10}: echocardiographic study," *Mol. Aspects Med.* 15 (1994): 149-54.

11. Murray, R.P., "Vitamin B_4: Missing Link to Cardiac Health" in *Nutritional Insights-1*, Shayne, V., ed, (1999).

12. Murray, M.T., *Encyclopedia of Nutritional Supplements* (Prima Publishing, 1996).

13. Sturman,J.A., "Nutritional taurine and central nervous system development," *Ann. N.Y. Acad. Sci.* 477 (1986): 196-213.

14. Huxtable, R.J., "Physiological actions of taurine," *Physiol. Rev.* 72 (1992): 101-63.

15. Jacobson, J.G., and Smith, L.H., "Biochemistry and physiology of taurine and taurine derivatives," *Physiol. Rev.* 48 (1968): 429-511.

16. Nara, Y., et al., "Effects of dietary taurine in blood pressures in spontaneously hypertensive rats," *Biochem. Pharmacol.* 27 (1978): 2689-92.

17. Azuma,J., et al., "Usefulness of taurine in chronic congestive heart failure and its prospective application," *Jpn. Circ. J.* 56 (1992): 95-99.

18. Chazov, E.I., et al., "Taurine and electrical activity of the heart," *Circ. Res.* 35 (1974): 11-21.

19. Hong, C.Y., et al., "Astragalus membranaceus and polygonum multiflorum protect rat heart," *Circa. Res.* 35 (1974): 11-21.

20. Li, S.Q., et al., "Clinical observation in the treatment of ischemic heart disease with astragalus membranaceus," *Chung Kuo, Chung Hsi, I. Chieh* 15 (1995): 77-80.

21. Xu, J.M., and Zheng, H.J., "Testing Sixty-four Patients with Arrhythmias by Ningxinbao capsules: A randomized, double-blind observation," *Shanghai J. of Trad. Chi. Med.* 4 (1994): 4-5.

22. Chen, D.G., "Effects of Jinshuibao Capsules on the Quality of Life of Patients with Heart Failure," *J. of Admin. of Trad. Chin. Med.* 5 (1995): 40-43.

23. "Cratagus—More than the heart? Part I," *Medi Herb Newsletter* no. 26-27 (1991).

24. Leuchtgens, H., "Crataegus Special Extract WS 1442 in NYHA II heart failure. A placebo- controlled randomized double-blind study," *Fortschr. Med.* 111 (1993): 352-54.

25. Schussler, M., et al., "Myocardial effects of flavonoids from crataegus species," *Arzneimitteiforschung* 45 (1995): 842-45.

26. Auguet, M., et al., "The pharmacological bases for the vascular impact of gingko biloba extract" in *Rokan (Ginkgo biloba). Recent results in pharmacology and clinic,* Funfgeld, E.W., ed. (New York: 1988): 169-79.

CHAPTER 13

1. Padrid, P., "Feline asthma: pathophysiology and treatment," *Waltham Focus* 9, no. 1 (1999).

2. Ibid.

3. Britton, J., "Dietary magnesium, lung function, wheezing, and airways and hyper-reactivity in a random adult population sample," *Lancet* 344 (1994): 357-62.

4. Kadrabova, J., et al., "Selenium status is decreased in patients with intrinsic asthma," *Biological Trace Element Research* 52 (1996): 241-48.

5. Hodge, L., et al., "Consumption of oily fish and childhood asthma risk," *J. Asthma* 22 (1996): 137-40.

6. Hatch, G.E., "Asthma: inhaled oxidants and dietary antioxidants," *Am. J. Clin. Nutr.* 61 (1995): 625-30.

7. Olusi, S.O., et al., "Plasma and white blood cell ascorbic acid concentration in patients with bronchial asthma," *Clinica chimca acta* 92 (1979): 161-66.

8. Reynolds, R.D., and Natta, C.L., "Depressed plasma pyridoxal phosphate concentrations in adult asthmatics," *Am. J. Clin. Nutr.* 41 (1985): 684-88.

9. Bartel, P.R., et al., "Vitamin B$_6$ supplementation and theophylline-related effects in humans," *Am. J. Clin. Nutr.* 60 (1994): 93-99.

10. Seamon, K.B., and Daly, J.W., "Forskolin: a unique diterpene activator of cyclic AMP-generating systems," *J. of Cyclic Nutr. Res.* 7 (1981): 201-24.

11. Wong, S., et al., "Forskolin inhibits platelet activating factor binding to platelet receptors independently of adenyl cyclase activation," *Eur. J. of Pharm.* 245 (1993): 51-61.

12. Kreutner, R.W., et al., "Bronchodilator and antiallergy activity of forskolin," *Eur. J. of Pharmacol.* 111 (1985): 1-8.

13. Tsunoo, A., et al., "Pharmacological Effects of the Mycelial Extract of Cultured Cordyceps Sinensis on Airways and Aortae of the Rat," proceedings of the 14th International Congress on the Science and Cultivation of Edible Fungi, Oxford, England, September 17-22, 1995.

14. Gilman, A.G., et al., *The Pharmacologic Basis of Therapeutics* (New York: MacMillan Publishing, 1980).

15. Wilkens, J.H., et al., "Effects of a PAF-antagonist (BN 52063) on broncho-constriction and platelet activation during exercise induced asthma," *Br. J. Clin. Pharmacol.* 29 (1990): 85-91.

16. Guinot, P., et al., "Effects of BN 52063, a specific PAF-acether antagonist on bronchial provocation test to allergens in asthmatic patients: A preliminary study," 34 (1987): 723-31.

17. Okimasu, E., et al., "Inhibitor of phospholipase A2 and platelet aggregation by glycyrrhizin, an anti-inflammatory drug," *Acta. Med. Okayama* 37 (1983): 385-91.

18. Macrides, T.A., et al., "The anti-inflammatory effects of omego-3-tetraenoic fatty acids isolated from a lipid extract (Lyprinol) from the New Zealand green-lipped mussel," Am oil chema Soc. Annual Meeting. Seattle, Washington, May 1997

19. Kim, H., et al., "Ginsenosides protect pulmonary vascular endothelium against free radical-induced injury," *Bioch. and Bioph. Res. Comm.* 189, no. 2 (1992): 670-76.

20. Gopalakrishnan, C., et al., "Effects of Tylophorine, a major alkaloid of tylophorine, a major alkaloid of tylophora indica, on immunopatholoigcal inflammatory reactions," *Ind. J. Med. Res.* 71 (1980): 940-48.

CHAPTER 14

1. Voith, V.L., and Borchelt, P.L., "Separation anxiety in dogs," *Comp. Contin. Educat. Pract. Vet.* 7, no. 4 (1985): 42-53.

2. "Pet Owner Survey," All Points Research (February 1997).

3. Houpt, K.A., et al., "Breaking the human-companion animal bond," *JAVMA* 208 (1996): 1653-57.

4. Miller, D.D., et al., "Factors associated with the decision to surrender a pet to an animal shelter," *JAVMA* 209 (1996): 738-42.

5. Simpson, B.S., and Simpson, D.M., "Behavioral Pharmacotherapy," in Voith, V.L., and Borchelt, P.L., ed., *Readings in Companion Animal Behavior First Edition* (Trenton, NJ: Vet. Learn. Syst., 1996): 100-15.

6. Kowalchik, C., and Hylton, W., ed., *Rodale's Illustrated Encyclopedia of Herbs* (Emmaus, PA: Rodale Press, 1987).

7. Wren, R.C., *Potter's New Cyclopedia of Botanical Drugs and Preparations* (Saffron Walden: C.W. Daniel Company Ltd., 1988): 201.

8. Davies, Gaba, et al., "Kava Pyrones and Resin: Studies on benzodiazepine binding sites in rodent brain," *Pharmacol. Toxicol.* 71 (1992): 120-26.

9.   Gleitz, J., et al., "Anticonvulsive action of (+/-) kavain estimated from its properties on stimulated synaptosomes and not channel receptor sites," *Eur. J. Pharmacol.* 315 (1996): 89-97.

10. Volz, H.P., and Kieser, M., "Kava kava extract WS 1490 versus placebo in anxiety disorders—a randomized placebo-controlled 25-week outpatient trial," *Pharmacopsychiatry* 30 (1997): 1-5.

11. Perovic, S., et al., "Pharmacological profile of hypericum extract," *Arzein-Forsch* 45 (1995): 1145-48.

12. Bladt, S., and Wagner, H., "Inhibition of MAO by fractions and constituents of hypericum extract," *J. Geriatric. Psychiatry Neurol.* 7 (1994): 557-59.

13. Mennini, T., et al., "In vitro study on the interaction of extracts and pure compounds from Valariana officinalis roots with GABA, benzodiazepine and barbituate receptors in rat brain," *Fitoterapia* 54 (1993): 291-300.

14. Milgram, N.W., et al., "Cognitive functions and aging in the dog: Acquisition of nonspatial visual tasks," *Behavioral Neurosci.* 108, no. 1 (1994): 57-69.

15. Gerlach, M., et al., "Effects of disease and aging on monoamine oxidase A and B," in *Monoamine Oxidase Inhibitors in Neurological Diseases,* Lieberman, A., Olanow, C.W., Youdini, M.B.H., and Tipton, K., eds. (New York: Marcel Dekker, 1994): 21-30.

16. Weiss, G.B., "Metabolism and actions of CDP-choline as an endogenous compound and administered exogenously as citicoline," *Life Sci.* 56 (1995): 637-60.

17. Cacabelos, R., et al., "Therapeutic effects of CDP-choline in Alzheimer's disease: Cognition, brain mapping, cerebrovascular hemodynamics and immune factors," *Ann. N.Y. Acad. Sci.* 777 (1996): 399-403.

18. Drago, F., et al., "Effects of cytidine-diphosphocholine on acetylcholine-mediated behaviors in the rat," *Brain Res. Bull.* 31 (1993): 485-89.

19. Petkov, V.D., et al., "Effects of CDP-choline on learning and memory processes in rodents," *Methods Find Exp. Clin. Pharmical.* 14 (1992): 593-605.

20. Knoll, J., "Longevity study with (-) Deprenyl," *Mech. of Aging and Develop.* 45 (1988): 237-62.

21. Milgram, M., "Maintenance of L-Deprenyl Prolongs Life in Aged Male Rats," *Life Sciences* 47 (1990): 415-20.

22. Knoll, J., "Longevity study with (-) Deprenyl," *Mech. of Aging and Develop.* 45 (1988): 237-62.

23. Tattons, W.G., et al., "Deprenyl Reduces PC12 Apoptosis by Inducing New Protein Synthesis," *Journal of Neurochemistry* 63 (1994): 1572-75.

24. Kanowski, S., et al., "Proof of the Efficacy of the Ginkgo biloba Special Extract Egb 761 in outpatients suffering from mild to moderate primary degenerative dementia of the Alzheimer Type of Multi-Infarct Dementia," *Phytomedicine* 4 (1997): 3-13.

25. Ogane, N. et al., "Effects of MS muscarinic receptor agonist on the central cholinergic system, evaluation by brain microdialysis," *Neuroscience Letter* 114 (1990): 55-100.

26. Crook, T., et al., "Effects of phosphatidylserine in Alzheimer's disease," *Psychopharmacal. Bull.* 28 (1992): 61-66.

27. Kiss, B., and Karpati, E., "Mechanisms of action of Vinpocetine," *Acta. Pharm. Hung.* 66, no. 5 (1996): 213-24.

28. Faloon, W., "Staying Mentally Sharp: European "Smart Drug" Now a Dietary Supplement," *Life Extension* (December 1998).

29. Hagiwara, H., et al., "Effect of Vinpocetine (TCV-3B) on cyclic GMP metabolism," *Folia Pharmacal. Japan* 80 (1982): 317-23.

30. Cruz, J., *Neurologic and Neurological Emergencies* (Philadelphia: W.B. Saunders Co., 1998): 51-88.

31. Dharmananda, S., *Gastrodia* (Portland, OR: Institute for Traditional Medicine, April 1998).

32. Booth, H., "Present Day Status of the Vitamins," *Lancet* 57, no. 12 (December 1937): 531.

33. Elvehjem, C.A., "Vitamin B Fractions, Their Nomenclature and Their Functions," *Journal of Nutrition* 13, no. 6 (June 10, 1937): 11.

34. Clemmons, R.M., "Degenerative myelopathy," *Veterinary Clinics of North America* 22 (1992): 965-71.

35. Goldsmith, H.S., "Omental transposition to the brain for Alzheimer's disease," *Ann. N.Y. Acad. Sci.* 826 (1997): 323.

36. Goldsmith, H.S., "Omental Transposition for Alzheimer's disease," *Neurol. Res.* 18 (1996): 103.

37. Goldsmith, H.S., "Brain and spinal cord revascularization by Omental transposition," *Neurol. Res.* 16 (1994): 159.

38. Goldsmith, H.S., et al., "Axonal regeneration after spinal cord transection and reconstruction," *Brain Res.* 589 (1999): 217.

39. Goldsmith, H.S., et al., "Omentum transposition for cerebral infraction: a thirteen-year follow-up study," *Surg. Neural.* 51 (1999): 342.

40. Goldsmith, H.S., et al., "Increased vascular perfusion after administration of an omentum lipid fraction," *Surg. Gynecal. Abstet.* 162 (1986): 579.

41. Ohtaki, T., et al., "Purification of acidic fibroblast growth factor from bovine omentum," *Biochem. Biopys. Res. Commun.* (1989): 161-69.

CHAPTER 15

1. Bronson, R.T., "Variation in age at death of dogs of different sexes and breeds," *Am. J. Vet. Res.* 43 (1982): 2057-59.

2. Lin, D.J., *Free Radicals and Disease Prevention* (Keats Publishing, Inc., 1953).

3. Issels, J., *Cancer: Second Opinion* (London: Hodder and Stoughton, 1987).

4. Reiter, R.J., et al., "A review of the evidence supporting melatonin's role as an antioxidant," *J. Pineal. Res.* 18, no. 1 (1995): 1-11.

5. Ames, B.N., et al., "Oxidants, antioxidants and the degenerative disease of aging," *Proc. Natl. Acad. Sci. Septe.* 90 (1993): 7915-22.

6. Bigelsen, H., "Treating Cancer," *Health Freedom News* 12, no. 8 (1993): 26-28.

7. Lynes, B., *The Healing of Cancer* (Marcus Books, 1989).

8. Quillin, P., *Beating Cancer with Nutrition* (Tulsa, OK: Nutrition Times Press, Inc., 1998).

9. Hayes, H.M., Tarone, R.E., and Cantor, K.P., et al., "Case control study of canine malignant lymphoma: Positive association with dog owner's use of 2,4 - dichlorophenoxyacetic acid herbicides," *J. Natl. Cancer Inst.* 83 (1998): 1226-31.

10. Pennisi, E., "New Gene Forges Link Between Fragile Site and Many Cancers," *Science* 272, no. 5263 (May 1996): 649.

11. King, M.C., et al., "Inherited Breast and Ovarian Cancer," *J.A.M.A.* 269, no. 15 (April 21, 1993).

12. Issels, J., *Cancer: Second Opinion* (London: Hodder and Stoughton, 1987).

13. Valentine, Tom, "Good News for Red Meat Gourmands," *Search for Health* 2, no. 425 (March/June 1994).

14. Ginsberg, R.J., et al., "Cancer of the lung," in DeVita, *Cancer Principles and Practices of Oncology* (Philadelphia: Lippincott, 1993).

15. Faloon, W., "Using Arthritis Drugs to Treat Cancer," *Life Extension* (February 2000).

16. Todorov., D.K., et al., "Antitumor Activity of Dionae Muscpula E. Carnivora new in vitro and in vivo on animal and human tumors," *Biotechnical. & Biotechnical. Eq.* (December 1998).

17. Walker, M., "Conquering Cancer at the Bavarian Klinik Winnerhof," *Townsend Letter for Doctors and Patients* (August/September 1999).

18. Kreher, B., et al., "Structure elucidation of Plumbagin-analogues from Dionea muscipala and their immunomodulating activities in vitro and in vivo," *Hungarian Chen. Soc. Int. Symp.* (August 1999).

19. Wrba, H., "New Approaches in Treatment of Cancer with Enzymes," First International Conference on Systemic Enzymes Therapy (September 12, 1990).

20. Thomas, R., *The Essiac Report* (Los Angeles: Alternative Treatment Information Network, 1993).

21. Moss, R., *Cancer Therapy: The Independent Consumer's Guide to Nontoxic Treatment and Prevention* (New York: Equinox Press, 1992).

22. Chen, Q.H., et al., "Studies on Chinese Rhubarb: Effect of Anthraquinone Derivatives on the Respiration and Glycolysis of Ehrlich Ascites Carcinoma Cells," *Acts Pharmaceutica Sinica* 15 (1980): 65-70.

23. Lu, M., and Chen, Q.H., "Biochemical Study of Chinese Rhubarb: Inhibitory Effects of Arthraquinone Derivatives on P 338 Leukemia in Mice," *J. of China Pharm. University* 20 (1989): 155-57.

24. Morita, K., et al., "A Desmutagenic Factor isolated from Burdoch (arctium lappa limme)," *Mutation Research* 129 (1984): 25-31.

25. Jones, K., *Pau d'Arco: Immune Power from the Rain Forest* (Vermont: Healing Arts Press, 1995).

26. Santana, C.F., et al., "Preliminary Observations with the Use of Lapachol in Human Patients Bearing Malignant Neoplasms," cited in Werbach, M.R., and Murray, M.T., *Botanical Influences on Illness* (Tarzara, CA: Third Line Press, 1994).

27. Gunther, E., *Ethnobotony of Western Washington: The knowledge and use of indigenous plants by Native Americans* (Seattle and London: Lewis of Wash. Press, 1992).

28. Christy, M.M., *The Pacific Yew Story. How an Ancient Tree Became a Modern Miracle* (Scottsdale, AZ: Wishland Publishing, 1999).

index

About the Author

Henry Pasternak, D.V.M., C.V.A., has practiced integrative medicine, using both holistic and Western therapies, at the Highlands Veterinary Hospital in Pacific Palisades, California, since 1990. He has a doctor's degree in veterinary medicine from the University of Missouri–Columbia and is certified in veterinary acupuncture by the International Veterinary Acupuncture Society. He is a member of the Holistic Veterinary Medical Association, the California Veterinary Medical Association, the Southern California Veterinary Medical Association, and the American Animal Hospital Association. Dr. Pasternak has studied holistic medicine with experts in China and the United States. Dr. Henry Pasternak is available for phone consultation (310-454-2917) for difficult-to-treat or life-threatening diseases.

Quick Order Form

Telephone orders: Call 310-454-2917. Have your credit card ready.

Fax orders: 310-454-3412. Send this form.

For online orders and more information:
Please visit www.petholisticare.com

Postal orders:
Highlands Veterinary Hospital
526 Palisades Drive
Pacific Palisades, CA 90272

Name _____

Address _____

City _____ State _____ Zip _____

Country _____

Telephone _____

E-mail address _____

Sales tax: Please add 8% for books shipped.

Shipping and handling:
In United States: $5.00 for the first book & $3.00 for each additional book
International: $10.00 for the first book & $6.00 for each additional book

Payment: ❏ Check   ❏ Credit Card

        ❏ Visa   ❏ MasterCard   ❏ Discover

Card Number _____

Name on card _____

Expiration date _____